Leisure and Everyday Life
with Dementia

Reconsidering Dementia Series Editors: Dr Keith Oliver and Professor Dawn Brooker MBE

Titles in the series

Dementia and Psychotherapy Reconsidered, Richard Cheston

Education and Training in Dementia Care: A Person-Centred Approach, Claire Surr, Sarah Jane Smith and Isabelle Latham

Dementia and Ethics Reconsidered, Julian C. Hughes

Leisure and Everyday Life with Dementia, Karen Gray, Christopher Russell and Jane Twigg (eds)

Forthcoming titles

Reconsidering Neighbourhoods and Living with Dementia: Spaces, Places, and People, John Keady (ed.)

Talking with Dementia, Reconsidered, Keith Oliver, Reinhard Guss and Ruth Bartlett

Leisure and Everyday Life with Dementia

Karen Gray, Christopher Russell and Jane Twigg

Open University Press

Open University Press
McGraw Hill
Unit 4,
Foundation Park
Roxborough Way
Maidenhead
SL6 3UD

email: emea_uk_ireland@mheducation.com
world wide web: www.openup.co.uk

First edition published 2024

Commissioning Editor: Sam Crowe
Editorial Assistant: Hannah Jones
Production Manager: Hannah Cartwright
Marketing Manager: Bryony Waters
Cover Design: Adam Renvoize
Cover Art: Jane Twigg
Logo Design: Julia Heron

A catalogue record of this book is available from the British Library

ISBN-13: 978-0-3352-5130-8
ISBN-10: 0335251307
eISBN: 978-0-3352-5131-5

Library of Congress Cataloging-in-Publication Data
CIP data applied for

Typeset by Transforma Pvt. Ltd., Chennai, India

Printed and bound by CPI Group (UK) Ltd, Croydon, CR0 4YY

Praise Page

"This exciting and unique book provides a significant collection of the research base and theory surrounding leisure and dementia. As described in one of the chapters, "People living with dementia described how leisure is an important way to celebrate living" – this view is certainly present throughout the book. It offers a contemporary understanding to leisure in the context of dementia, with thought-provoking examples that are perfect for guiding in-class discussions. It covers a diverse range of topics written by leading experts in the field, including people living with dementia, making it a must-have text for anyone working in the field of dementia care!"

Dr Mary O'Malley, BSc, PhD, CPsychol, Senior Research Fellow,
Association for Dementia Studies, University of Worcester, UK

"This is the most important edited collection to emerge from leisure studies in the last thirty years. The evidence across the chapters shows the crucial role leisure plays in the everyday lives and wellbeing of people living with dementia, their families and others around them. This book is a vital resource for policymakers in health and social care, professionals, and academics interested in the intersection of leisure and health and wellbeing."

Professor Karl Spracklen, School of Humanities and Social Sciences,
Leeds Beckett University, UK

"This book is a 'must' read for anyone working or supporting someone who has had a dementia diagnosis. Indeed, it may offer many new ideas for leisure for those living with dementia. Combining theory and practical solutions, much of the learning involving social citizenship wider than friends and family in the supporting of people living with dementia to increase activity or remain active through leisure is vital for an enriched quality of life and better physical, mental and social health outcomes. The multidisciplinary viewpoints but also the involvement of Jane Twigg, living with a diagnosis of dementia, brought the words to life and ensured resonance with those that will benefit. Mostly, it shows that choice and preferences, freedom and support to do what they want to do, when they want to do it, should always be central to supporting meaningful leisure opportunities."

Professor Dawn Skelton, Professor of Ageing & Health, Glasgow
Caledonian University, UK and Chair of the British Geriatrics
Society Rehabilitation Group

"This edited book shifts perspectives by focussing on leisure, an area that dementia studies seldom address. 'Living with dementia' is a phrase used more widely as the number of people affected by the diagnosis increases, but the phrase begs many questions. Living well or miserably? Surviving or thriving? Feeling in control or overburdened? Contented or depressed? Leisure is important because most people with dementia are not in employment. For them – as for the general population past working age, leisure a major determinant of wellbeing. This timely collection opens up new avenues of thought and research for all those concerned with the quality of life of people with dementia."

Justine Schneider, Professor of Mental Health and Social Care, School of Sociology & Social Policy, University of Nottingham, UK

"'Leisure and Everyday Life with Dementia' is a novel collection of works that not only broadens and enriches our understandings of the importance of leisure for people living with dementia, but in demonstrating the possibilities for living well with dementia through engagement with leisure, it helps to build the foundation for developing an ethical standard to support such engagement to the fullest extent possible."

Pia Kontos, Senior Scientist and Professor, KITE Research Institute, Toronto Rehabilitation Institute – University Health Network, and Dalla Lana School of Public Health, University of Toronto, Canada

"This book makes an important contribution to understanding and navigating how those with dementia can live well with the condition. With contributions by a diverse group of scholars, practitioners and those with dementia, an impressive array of approaches, activities and ideas are proposed, supported by research evidence. The practical guidance included means that the book will be valuable for those living with dementia, their supporters and health and social care staff. The text demonstrates that leisure time, whether it involves walking, participating in sport, or listening to music is not simply a nice diversion but that it truly makes life worth living."

Professor Victoria Tischler, University of Surrey, UK

Contents

About the editors

Dr Karen Gray: Karen is a researcher at the University of Bristol (UK) with wide-ranging experience in researching and evaluating engagement in arts, creativity and physical activity for health and well-being. She has a particular interest in how we understand and value these activities and the methodologies we use to do this. Karen holds a first doctorate in literature and a second (funded by the Alzheimer's Society) that explored the challenges of evaluating arts activities for people living with dementia.

Dr Chris Russell: Chris is a senior lecturer with the Association for Dementia Studies at the University of Worcester (UK), where he is Programme Lead for the Postgraduate Certificate in Dementia Studies. His research focuses on the experiences of leisure for people living with dementia, in particular when engaging in physical activity. A qualified social worker, Chris also has a keen interest in social citizenship for people living with dementia. He has completed research and published on this topic – for example, exploring the contribution of people living with dementia to teaching in higher education.

Jane Twigg: Jane's background is as a physiotherapist. This was before caring for her Mom, who had dementia, including supporting Mom to continue to live in the world. Jane is now living with atypical dementia. She has a passion for life. Long distance walking brings her most joy, giving her a sense of achievement and well-being.

Contributors

Dr Ruth Bartlett: School of Health Sciences, University of Southampton (UK) and Faculty of Health Studies, VID Specialized University (Norway)

Zoe Estelle Brown: PhD candidate in Adult Nursing, University of Northumbria (UK)/Outreach Officer, Culture, Health and Communities, Tyne & Wear Archives & Museums (UK)

Dr Liz Carlin: Lecturer, Division of Sport and Exercise, University of the West of Scotland (UK)

Dr Jennifer Carson: Director, Dementia Engagement, Education and Research (DEER) Program, School of Public Health, University of Nevada, Reno (USA)

Joanne Charlton: Platinum Programme Lead, Tyne & Wear Archives & Museums (UK)

Prof Helen Chatterjee: Professor of Human and Ecological Health, UCL Biosciences/UCL Arts and Sciences, University College London (UK)

Dr Robyn Dowlen: Research Associate, Division of Nursing, Midwifery and Social Work, University of Manchester (UK)

Dr Becky Dowson: Research Fellow, School of Sociology and Social Policy and Institute of Mental Health, University of Nottingham (UK)/Music Therapist, Chiltern Music Therapy (UK)

Dr Sherry Dupuis: Professor and University Research Chair, Department of Recreation and Leisure Studies, University of Waterloo (Canada)

Dr Shirley Evans: Senior Research Fellow, Association for Dementia Studies, University of Worcester (UK)

Dr Simon Evans: Principal Research Fellow, Association for Dementia Studies, University of Worcester (UK)

Dr Darla Fortune: Associate Professor, Department of Applied Human Sciences, Concordia University (Canada)

Dr Rebecca Genoe: Professor, Faculty of Kinesiology and Health Studies, University of Regina (Canada)

Dr Karen Gray: Senior Research Associate, School for Policy Studies, University of Bristol (UK)

Brenda Hounam: Dementia Advocate and Co-Researcher, Living and Celebrating Life through Leisure Project (Canada)

Dr Anthea Innes: Professor of Health, Aging and Society, Gilbrea Chair in Aging and Mental Health, Director Gilbrea Centre for Studies in Aging, McMaster University (Canada)

Prof John Keady: Professor of Mental Health Nursing and Older People and Senior Fellow, NIHR School for Social Care Research, Division of Nursing, Midwifery and Social Work, University of Manchester/Greater Manchester Mental Health NHS Foundation Trust (UK)

Claire Linton: Department of Health Sciences, Lakehead University (Canada)

Dr Eilidh Macrae: Senior Lecturer, Division of Sport and Exercise, University of the West of Scotland (UK)

Dr Rhoda Macrae: Reader, Alzheimer Scotland Centre for Policy and Practice, Division of Mental Health and Integrated Practice, University of the West of Scotland (UK)

Carlina Marchese: Knowledge Broker, Centre for Education and Research on Aging and Health, Lakehead University (Canada)

Nancy McAdam: Dementia Advocate, Member of Scottish Dementia Alumni DEEP Group, Person Living with Dementia (UK)

Sophie Mitchell: Outreach Officer, Culture, Health and Communities, Tyne & Wear Archives & Museums (UK)

Dr Nuala Morse: Lecturer in Museum Studies, School Museum Studies, University of Leicester (UK)

Dr Rebecca Oatley: Lecturer, School of Social Sciences, Cardiff University (UK)

Dr Chris Russell: Lecturer, Association for Dementia Studies, University of Worcester (UK)

Dr Robert A. Stebbins: Professor Emeritus, Department of Sociology, University of Calgary (Canada)

Dr Nisha Sutherland: Associate Professor, School of Nursing, Lakehead University (Canada)

Dr Juliana Thompson: Associate Professor in Adult Nursing, Northumbria University (UK)

Jane Twigg: Lived experience of dementia, Worcestershire (UK)

Bailey Vandorp: Research Assistant, Department of Health Sciences, Lakehead University (Canada)

Dr Joseph Webb: Lecturer, School for Policy Studies, University of Bristol (UK)

Dr Joy Watson: Dementia Advocate, Ambassador with the Alzheimer's Society, Associate with 3 Nations Dementia Working Group, Person Living with Dementia (UK)

Lindsay Watt: Department of Health Sciences, Lakehead University (Canada)

Dr Elaine Wiersma: Associate Professor, Department of Health Sciences/ Associate Director, Centre for Education and Research on Aging & Health, Lakehead University (Canada)

Colleen Whyte: Associate Professor, Department of Recreation and Leisure Studies, Brock University (Canada)

Forewords

Hopes and reflections

Jane Twigg

My hope for this book is that those reading it will learn the importance of listening to people like me who are living with a diagnosis of dementia – to involve and include us in a safe and supportive environment, finding our way to enjoy leisure (whatever that means to us as individuals), being in the moment, with choice and communication at its heart.

The importance of any leisure activity for me is that it must be life-enhancing.

I was pleased to have been invited to work as an editor, because I like a challenge! It gave me the opportunity to contribute to something significant – such as this book on leisure – about people living with dementia. It feels of value to me, to give a perspective from someone living with a diagnosis, who has lived experience. This has only been made possible by having support to help facilitate the process.

So how did we work? The person supporting assisted me by reading each dementia-friendly summary out loud, and slowly, while I listened with my eyes closed. Closing my eyes cuts out distractions and allows me to focus. This process is important, as while I can read myself, having it read out loud allows me to absorb the words and understand what has been written, rather than the words disappearing off the page, without real meaning. Working in this way allowed us to explore together what had been written and helped me to clarify my thoughts and feelings, which my support was then able to document, for us to fine-tune later. This was a lengthy process of refining, sentence by sentence, to give feedback. Key to this way of working was having a great, established relationship, already in place, from someone who has known me well over several years. I was fortunate enough to have assistance from this person, who I had previously worked with and who kindly volunteered her time, otherwise there would have been a financial implication, with me having to fund support to take up the opportunity.

Due to the pandemic, my support and I have needed to work remotely when editing the summaries, which was an added challenge, as we normally work face to face. We have also met regularly with one of the other editors on Zoom, which has worked really well, and to have had the reassurance that I/we were on track with what was required, was also very helpful. I also had the opportunity to meet with some of the authors via Zoom. Feedback from them on my contribution has left me feeling listened to and included. It has also been of great value to work in partnership with the two other editors to influence the publishers to look at the contractual issues in writing a book and ensure they are dementia-friendly.

Being an editor has been a bigger commitment than I had anticipated. However, I am glad to have had this opportunity to work as an editor, as it has been a huge privilege.

Leisure and dementia

Robert A. Stebbins

This book is an exciting prospect. Dementia and leisure combine to form a distinctive human condition, and one that is largely neglected in the study of leisure and in wider society. This is the first time, for example, that an edited collection on dementia and leisure has been published.

Leisure is a wide-ranging and diverse discipline, and several significant theories come to mind, with potential relevance to the book's subject matter – for example, therapeutic recreation (TR), the branch of this field that focuses directly on a person's rehabilitation and adaptation available through leisure. Such recreation has mostly centred on physical and cognitive disabilities for which appropriate leisure activities can offer significant rehabilitation and adaptation. However, might TR be applied to the dementia context? Certainly, its emphasis on the friends and family of the person, and the wider community and social world to which people with disabilities belong, resonates with a theme of this book: social citizenship. The focus on social citizenship fits well, because it is the collective of the person, their family and professionals that is often required to promote the best outcomes for individuals.

Serious leisure is the regular pursuit of an amateur, hobbyist or volunteer – activity that people find so substantial, interesting and fulfilling that, in the typical case, they launch themselves on a (leisure) career centred on acquiring and expressing a combination of its special skills, knowledge and experience. Might the chapters which follow shed light on ways in which people living with dementia exercise serious leisure?

Casual leisure, meanwhile, is an immediately, naturally rewarding, relatively short-lived, pleasurable activity, requiring little or no special training to enjoy it. It is pursued for its significant level of pure enjoyment, or pleasure. Examples range from observing scenery, to playing a board game using dice, or serving as a volunteer. It can include sociable conversation, a type of casual leisure that may well be universal. All societies seem to have places where, and occasions during which, members gossip, tell jokes, discuss the weather and banter (josh, engage in repartee). Telling anecdotes and reminiscing are also lively components of this kind of leisure. The most satisfying of such social citizenship is when it is face to face, even while circumstances may force participants to use a telephone or, nowadays, Zoom or Skype. Some of the casual activities of the sensory stimulation kind described earlier are also relaxing. Additionally, walks in natural settings like wooded areas and areas featuring creeks, rivers and lakes can be enjoyable. Bus tours offer such stimulation available in more distant sites. Finally, access to a pet falls into this class of casual leisure.

Project-based leisure is a short-term, moderately complicated, either one-shot or occasional, though infrequent, creative undertaking carried out in free time. It requires planning, effort, and sometimes skill or knowledge, but for all that is neither serious leisure nor intended by the participant to develop into such. It is a leisure project when we volunteer to help out at an arts festival or sports event, develop the basement at home, or arrange a big celebration for a fiftieth wedding anniversary, assuming that these are not recurrent activities for us. As with serious and casual leisure it is carried out in free time, or time unhampered by disagreeable obligations; this arouses further curiosity about matters that might be considered within this collection. How much free time do people living with dementia have, how far is this even considered, and how often might it be impeded by the routines of formalized care?

These are the kinds of activities and questions that rise to the fore when considering the collection contained within this book. Its chapters serve to demonstrate some of the ways in which people living with dementia could be enabled to continue or take up leisure activities – and how they and society might benefit from this.

Citizenship and dementia

Ruth Bartlett

The field of dementia studies has come a long way in the last thirty years. At one time, academic debates about people living with dementia revolved around person-centred care and therapies. Nowadays, discussions have expanded to include everyday life and disability rights. This broadening of scope and practice has opened new avenues of research, and more importantly helped to bring the ordinary (as opposed to medical) lives of people living with dementia into keener focus. It is a development that provokes one to consider how well we are doing as a society in terms of enabling people living with dementia to participate in everyday life on an equal basis with others.

This book brings together a strong collection of works about the participation of people with dementia in leisure activities. The chapters are organized around three sections or realms of everyday life, which I see in this way: ethical – why people engage in leisure activities; practical – how people engage; and locational – where people engage. The framing allows for rich stories to be told about leisure, including the meaning of leisure to people living with dementia; the pleasures and challenges of participating in different sports, such as badminton and walking football; tourism and the travel industry; listening to music; being outside in nature; visiting museums and spending time online. Each chapter explores the topic from the perspective of people living with dementia and in the context of the latest thinking about living a good life with dementia. Freedom is a strong theme running through the entire text.

As a scholar with a long-standing interest in broadening the lens to include the everyday lives of people with living with dementia, and someone who enjoys her free time, I really am thrilled to see a text that focuses on leisure. It shows how far we have come as a research field, and how much more there is to do in terms of both awareness-raising and knowledge development. The stories in *Leisure and Everyday Life with Dementia* serve as a useful barometer for how well we are doing, particularly in respect of Article 30 of the United Nations Convention on the Rights of Persons with Disabilities, and social citizenship more broadly – not least because the text focuses on the perspectives of people living with dementia.

Article 30 of the Convention is about 'participation in cultural life, recreation, leisure, and sport'. It obligates those nation states who have signed up to the Convention to encourage and promote the participation, to the fullest extent possible, of people with disabilities in mainstream leisure activities at all levels. This book provides examples of the participation of people living with dementia in both ordinary and specialist leisure activities in the UK and Canada. As such, it represents what is currently possible for people living with dementia in these countries. It is important to have this collection, for leisure to develop as an area of inquiry in dementia studies. Article 30 also states (among other things) that nation states 'should take appropriate measures to enable persons with disabilities to have the opportunity to develop and utilize their creative, artistic and intellectual potential, not only for their own benefit, but also for the enrichment of society'. The ideas of 'creating the self' and 'in the moment' experiences, which are discussed in this book, signify a valuable way of enabling people with dementia to enjoy such opportunities. The works represented show us why it is so vital to keep broadening the debate and thinking about the everyday lives of citizens with dementia.

The Reconsidering Dementia Series

The dementia field has developed rapidly in its scope and practice over the past 25 years. Many thousands of people are newly diagnosed each year. Worldwide, the trend is that people are being diagnosed at much earlier stages. In addition, families and friends increasingly provide support to those affected by dementia over a prolonged period. Many people, both those diagnosed with dementia and those who support them, have an appetite to understand their condition. Care professionals and civic society also need an in-depth and nuanced understanding of how to support people living with dementia within their communities over the long term. The Reconsidering Dementia book series sets out to address this need. It takes its inspiration from the late Professor Tom Kitwood's seminal text *Dementia Reconsidered*, published in 1997, which, at the time, revolutionized how dementia care was conceptualized.

The book series is jointly commissioned and edited by Professor Dawn Brooker MBE and by Dr Keith Oliver. Dawn has been active in the field of dementia care since the 1980s as a clinician and an academic. She draws on her experience and international networks to bring together a series of books on the most pertinent issues in the field. Keith is one of the foremost international advocates for those living with dementia. He also brings an insightful perspective of his own and others' experience of what it means to live with dementia gained since his diagnosis of Alzheimer's disease in 2010.

Dawn and Keith have been professional colleagues for many years. They both worked together on the second edition of Kitwood's book, *Dementia Reconsidered, Revisited: The Person Still Comes First.* This 2019 publication was a reprint of the original text by Tom Kitwood alongside contemporary commentaries for each chapter written by current experts. Many topics in the field of dementia care, however, were simply unheard of in Kitwood's lifetime. When Open University Press approached Dawn and Keith with the idea of developing a book series dedicated to dementia, they were very pleased to accept. The subsequent titles in this series are cutting-edge scholarly texts that challenge and engage readers to think deeply. They draw on theoretical understandings, contemporary research and experience to critically reflect on their topic in great depth.

This does not mean, however, that they are not applicable to improving the care and support of those affected by dementia. As well as the scholarly text all books have a 'So what?' thread that unpacks what this means for people living with dementia, their families, people working in dementia care, policymakers, professionals, community activists and so on. Too many books either focus on an academic audience *or* a practitioner audience *or* a student audience *or* a lived experience audience. In this series, the aim is to try to address these perspectives in the round. The Reconsidering Dementia book series brings together the perspectives of professional practice, scholarship and lived experience as they pertain to the key topics in the field of dementia studies. All the books aim to help us to think afresh, to reconsider our standpoint and to ultimately improve the experience of those affected by dementia for years to come.

Preface

When Tom Kitwood first wrote *Dementia Reconsidered*, the idea that the concept of leisure would have any place in a book series on dementia would have been met with utter confusion. At the end of the last century, even the idea of using arts and music for therapeutic benefit was virtually unheard of. At best, it would have been seen as diversion or stimulation. The thought that people could enjoy leisure for its own sake was not a concept that would have been considered.

Twenty-five years on, thankfully, this idea is no longer radical. Many more people worldwide are now living with dementia and people are being diagnosed at much earlier stages. One of the advantages of this is that it provides the opportunity for people to incorporate living with dementia into their lives. How do we ensure that people can continue to enjoy activities and opportunities with friends old and new? We know that if people make good adjustments to life early on in their diagnosis, then they are likely to find it easier to cope with symptoms of dementia later on. However, many people continue to face unhelpful barriers from society and from professionals in this respect. The thinking around leisure and activity is often conflated with therapy interventions and treatments. Chris Russell and Karen Gray both tackled these ideas within their cutting edge PhD research. Together with Jane Twigg, they are very well placed to bring together an edited book that examines the concept of leisure in dementia from a multiplicity of angles. This is a far-reaching book which will be well read by many people from a whole range of backgrounds.

We hope that you will learn as much from it as we have.

Series editors: Dawn Brooker and Keith Oliver

Additional thoughts from Keith Oliver

When I was initially diagnosed with Alzheimer's disease aged 54 my wife and I were told by the neurologist to cancel a holiday to Australia. We did not do this, but slightly amended the itinerary and wrote to the neurologist to allay some of his concerns. He then gave his assent. We subsequently revisited Australia eight more times until the Covid-19 pandemic and our mutual health and ageing issues brought it to a (probable) close. Many people would have taken those words of the neurologist on board and wrapped themselves in a shroud of cotton wool, never enjoying what we have done since my diagnosis. Support, encouragement, opportunity and a little confidence is all one needs to enjoy many of the activities expertly outlined in this book.

I wholeheartedly commend this book to you, whether you are a professional working with people affected by dementia, someone working in one of the many aspects of leisure outlined in this book, an academic or a student, a person affected by dementia or an individual interested in the subject the book. There is something for you all to take from this, and if you do the lives of many of us will be much improved.

As a person who has lived with an Alzheimer's disease diagnosis and all that that has thrown at me and my wife for 12 years I see leisure as far more than having a good time, enjoying myself or even enhancing my well-being. I relate so closely to leisure in the ways described in this book, as the activities, places I visit and new and old connections to people, places and memories so enrich my life. For me, it simply makes my life worth living.

1 Considering leisure and dementia

Karen Gray and Chris Russell

Possibilities

We take part in leisure to enhance our lives. That guiding thought is returned to again and again throughout this book. A life enhanced is open to possibility, to purpose and to fun. It is also a life in which, through our own actions and in relationship with others, we might find ways to positively change our lives and those of other people.

That these possibilities are not equally open to people living with dementia is an injustice. In this book we seek to raise awareness of the role and meaning of leisure in the lives of people living with dementia, and to explore ways in which to tackle the injustice. We have deliberately addressed a broad readership. Our authors reflect different perspectives, practices and disciplines; some are themselves living with dementia.

'Nothing about us without us' (Bryden 2016) is what people living with dementia rightly demand, and this theme is fundamental to the book. In addition to authors living with dementia contributing to chapters, one of the editors, Jane Twigg, brings experience of everyday life with the syndrome. Jane's reflections on her role have been foregrounded at the start of the book, and they provide its vision, encouraging this to be about leisure being part of the everyday and life-affirming. The summaries that each author provides at the start of their chapters are intended to not only enhance the book's accessibility, they have also enabled Jane to play an active role in its development.

Understandings of dementia have changed radically over the past 30 years. There has been a marked shift from considering dementia as primarily a medical condition, to an understanding that it is something which affects all aspects of a person's experience of life. Key is the recognition that everybody's experience of dementia is different, and that we are all unique. Therefore, taking a person-centred approach means ensuring that each individual with dementia is recognized in terms of their life story, aptitudes and skills, personality and physical health, rather than being defined only by the cognitive impairment dementia has caused (Brooker and Latham 2016; Kitwood and Brooker 2019).

Yes, everyone is an individual, and everybody is different. There are also broader matters, however, influencing the experience of everyday life, that must be considered. For example, the gender (Sandberg 2018), ethnicity (Roche et al. 2020), sexuality (McParland and Camic 2018) and economic situation (Samuel et al. 2020) of people all play their part in the experience of everyday life for different individuals. These features, components of the structure upon which society is based, should not be disregarded simply because a person is living with dementia.

Personhood matters too – that is the relationships an individual living with dementia has with others, and the quality of those in terms of enabling that person to sustain their feeling of self and identity. This in turn links to social citizenship, a concept key to the collection included within this book. Social citizenship is the ability a person living with dementia has to sustain their place in the world and as an active participant in life, according to how they wish this to be (Bartlett and O'Connor 2007, 2010). As with personhood, realization of this will depend on the reactions and behaviour of others, and how comfortable individuals feel within the social environment where everyday life is played out and experienced. However, through social citizenship we recognize person-centred features, enabling relationships and opportunities to live a fulsome life, to be *rights* for people living with dementia, and not just optional extras. A person never ceases to be a citizen. It is not for others to deny this way of being based on a diagnosis of dementia. This is enshrined within the foundational principles of the United Nation's Universal Declaration of Human Rights and other international human rights instruments, in particular, as Ruth Bartlett has noted in her foreword, the Convention on the Rights of Persons with Disabilities (WHO 2021). There can be no 'us' and 'them'.

Leisure is a complex topic, with many definitions and potential ways to understand it. It may be understood differently around the world. In many countries leisure is a significant part of everyday life and is highly organized. Large sums of money are spent by individuals, organizations and charities on leisure and the structures that support it. And a great deal of research and scholarship has been and continues to be devoted to understanding it.

Some have argued that the notion of spare or free time is fundamental to leisure. In other words, it is what we, as individuals, choose to do when we have time. This inevitably raises the issue of work. Freedom from the obligations of work provides the time to engage in activities one wishes to. The picture is further complicated perhaps, because many people enjoy their work and engage in activities there which could be understood as leisure – for example, reading, taking exercise, gardening, dancing. Furthermore, the components of the structure of society, highlighted above, and economic circumstance in particular, will influence whether an individual is able to choose what they do in time that may be available to them. Freedom from domestic obligations, something that gives time to do other things, would seem a core requirement for leisure. Accordingly, we can see that choice is also a fundamental part of leisure, which must be about having the right and opportunity to choose what one does with the 'free' time one has.

The experiences of people living with dementia and their close family members, relating to leisure, have been explored only in relatively recent times. Several contributors to this book have led the way. Leisure is seen as important in the context of life with dementia largely because of some of the matters highlighted above – for example, freedom from obligations, and the ability to choose what one does with everyday life. In this way, therefore, leisure relates to the human rights and the citizenship of people affected by dementia.

Some of the theories that are applied to leisure are relevant for life with dementia in mind – for example, 'casual leisure' and 'serious leisure', both of which are introduced by leisure scholar Robert Stebbins (1997) in the first of our forewords. Another theory of leisure – 'communicative leisure' – explains how participating in leisure offers individuals the opportunity to strengthen their sense of identity. Fundamental to communicative leisure is interaction between participants; this provides the chance for exchange of ideas, and opportunities that maximize agency and the ability to make meaning from leisure activity. This also might afford opportunities for personal transformation, a space in which individuals make new meaning about themselves, and the building of new social networks (Spracklen 2013).

These theories help identify the value this book brings. Themes such as agency, choice, communality, collaboration, equality, fun and aspiration run through and across them. They also permeate and interweave with the understandings of person-centred and personhood approaches articulated earlier. Recognition of the social citizenship of individuals by others enables these foundational strands to be brought together. Precisely how this operates and what this means for people living with dementia is understanding that this book advances.

Because we want to think about leisure in the context of daily life with dementia and the ways in which participation in it enables people living with dementia to sustain their place in the world, we have structured this book into what we term the *realms of everyday life*.

Realm One: The individual, interactions and relationships

We take part in leisure as individuals, but also with and beside other people. This means that any consideration of our leisure participation must incorporate topics such as identity, rights, relationships and communication, as well as the individual and collective benefits we obtain from participation or demand if we are to have equal access to it. By attending to the meanings that people living with dementia might find in and through their individual experiences of leisure, we progress our understanding in these areas. Drawing on extensive research involving people living with dementia, Sherry Dupuis and her co-authors examine these meanings in the next chapter. They argue for a view of engagement in leisure as an opportunity for the continuation of interests, as well as for exploration, development, relaxation and for enjoyment of life. They present a novel framework for identifying how such opportunities might be enabled.

One of the key threads woven through this volume is that there is the potential for our attitudes towards leisure to be negatively affected by a prevailing focus on the value of leisure activity for its perceived therapeutic, or preventative, effects on the symptoms of dementia or its clinical progression. Several of our authors touch on this theme, including Becky Dowson, who explores concepts such as the 'musical self' and how people living with dementia feel about taking part in music alongside others, as part of an examination of the role that music can play in everyday life.

As we have already noted, leisure can offer people living with dementia the means to uphold existing identities outside their status as a person with the syndrome. However, inequalities linked to these identities can intersect with forms of discrimination inherent to dementia. Rebecca Oatley's chapter examines the issue through the lens of gender, taking the example of a sport reminiscence study and showing how assumptions about gender may interact with and influence leisure opportunities for people living with the condition.

Communication between people living with dementia and those who support their involvement in leisure can be crucial in enabling or impeding participation. Looking in detail at conversation taking place around facilitated group activities such as quizzes, Joseph Webb provides insight into how the voices of people living with dementia can be enabled or stifled by such interaction, but also how communication can help individuals to adapt or reshape participation and an activity itself according to their capacity or desire.

Realm Two: Time – how it is used and by whom

Contributors in this section focus on how people living with dementia engage in leisure and what factors could affect how they spend their time. The idea that people living with dementia might sustain their place in the world through their continued participation in everyday creative activity is central to Robyn Dowlen and John Keady's chapter. They suggest that an appreciation of 'in the moment' and 'here and now' experience in the context of music participation will provide insight helpful to those wishing to facilitate musical leisure opportunities for people living with dementia, as well as to researchers seeking to understand how to assess its true value beyond the therapeutic potential for those people taking part.

A regular game of badminton, a swim or a visit to a local gym could be beneficial to anybody's physical health, mental well-being or general happiness. However, doing these things is not always easy when you are living with dementia. The meaning and value of sustained everyday leisure participation, with physical activity as the focus, are topics progressed further by Chris Russell.

Opportunities for travel and holidays are a part of life for many of us, but they can be tricky to continue following a diagnosis of dementia. The vital and joyful perspectives and experiences of travelling and tourism of two co-authors who are living with dementia (Nancy McAdam and Joy Watson, working alongside researcher Anthea Innes) inform and are central to our next chapter.

Finally in this section, whether or not a person is able to make choices about these things can be affected by stigma, making it difficult for them to maintain a full and active involvement in the social world. Rebecca Genoe and her colleagues tackle this difficult topic head on. They argue for a view of leisure as a means of resisting preconceived ideas about loss and disability – offering instead a path to belonging and opportunities to explore strengths, capacity, and to experience well-being.

Realm Three: Place, places and spaces: their nature, use and meaning

Here we turn towards an examination of the locations, physical and virtual, indoor and outdoor, in which people living with dementia engage in leisure. Elaine Wiersma and her co-authors argue that certain kinds of leisure spaces provide opportunities for people to experience *freedom to be* and *freedom to do* – to feel they belong. This chapter explores the qualities, characteristics and facilitating factors for 'third places' – informal and inclusive public spaces where people living with dementia might enjoy casual socialization – through an investigation of an art programme and a dementia cafe.

Attitudes towards dementia and misunderstandings around risk mean that people living with dementia may find all kinds of indoor and outdoor spaces inaccessible. Underpinning a chapter from Simon Evans is the idea that connecting with outdoor spaces and with elements of the natural world is not only beneficial for well-being and helpful in sustaining a sense of belonging and community, but that opportunity and access to nature should itself be viewed as a human right.

Calling on a depth of knowledge from both museum practitioners and researchers, Nuala Morse and colleagues examine the role of accessible and inclusive museum spaces and programmes in supporting the active social citizenship of people living with dementia and in giving voice to their experiences through an engagement with museum collections. This is followed by Rhoda Macrae and her fellow contributors who examine how the welcoming environment of Scotland's national sports stadium, Hampden Park, shaped the experiences of people taking part in dementia-friendly walking football activities there.

Our ability to connect with the world outside our own four walls, and with other people, was curtailed by conditions widely experienced during Covid-19 lockdowns. Such deprivations were felt particularly keenly by many people living with dementia. The pandemic has accelerated appreciation of how important it is to ensure equality of participation within, and access to, online environments. Our final chapter in this section, co-authored by Shirley Evans and Jane Twigg, discusses the ways in which technology affords access to leisure, thereby promoting and enabling connectivity for people living with dementia, as well as the barriers that can impede such experience.

This is the first time that a collection of cutting-edge contemporary scholarship incorporating dementia and leisure has been published together. Contributors have been drawn from across disciplines and continents. Their chapters reference leisure activities ranging from the arts and culture, to sports and physical activity, to quizzes and games. Maintaining this breadth was important to us; we wanted it to be clear that no one kind of activity can be privileged over another. However, we could not cover everything and must acknowledge significant gaps. These include a pressing need to include the scholarship of those from wider international perspectives, and in particular the Global South, to explore what may be differing perspectives on leisure resulting from geography and culture, and to provide greater depth around this and other key intersectional issues.

One of the ways in which people living with dementia might potentially experience increased access to leisure provision is as a result of social prescribing. There is, so far, a lack of clarity about what this might involve and consistency in approach, but it tends to involve practitioners employed within primary healthcare who initiate participation in interventions designed to meet the social needs of individuals, with the aim of bringing about beneficial impacts on health and well-being (Sandhu et al. 2022). Welcome though this may be, the incorporation of leisure activities under the umbrella of social prescribing brings with it the risk that leisure becomes medicalized. While this book includes content that may be of use to those offering social prescription, it maintains an emphasis on leisure being a core part of everyday life.

We hope that this volume is just a start and that it will inspire further engagement with the subject, including through application of some of the recommendations and links to practice that authors have included. Supported by the 'So what does this mean in practice?' sections that end each of the following chapters, as you read on, we encourage you to reflect on and apply what you learn to enhance the lives of people affected by dementia.

References

Bartlett, R. and O'Connor, D. (2007) From personhood to citizenship: Broadening the lens for dementia practice and research, *Journal of Aging Studies*, 21(2): 107–18.

Bartlett, R. and O'Connor, D. (2010) *Broadening the Dementia Debate: Towards Social Citizenship*. Bristol: Policy Press.

Brooker, D. and Latham, I. (2016) *Person-Centred Dementia Care: Making Services Better with the VIPS Framework*, 2nd edn. London and Philadelphia: Jessica Kingsley Publishers.

Bryden, C. (2016) *Nothing About Us Without Us*. London: Jessica Kingsley Publishers.

Kitwood, T. and Brooker, D. (2019) *Dementia Reconsidered Revisited: The Person Still Comes First*. London: Open University Press.

McParland, J. and Camic, P.M. (2018) How do lesbian and gay people experience dementia?, *Dementia*, 17(4): 452–77.

Roche, M., Higgs, P., Aworinde, J. and Cooper, C. (2020) A review of qualitative research of perception and experiences of dementia among adults from Black, African, and

Caribbean background: What and whom are we researching?, *The Gerontologist*, 61(5): 195–208.

Samuel, L.J., Szanton, S.L., Wolff, J.L. et al. (2020) Socioeconomic disparities in six-year incident dementia in a nationally representative cohort of US older adults: An examination of financial resources, *BMC Geriatrics*, 20(1): 156.

Sandberg, L.J. (2018) Dementia and the gender trouble? Theorising dementia, gendered subjectivity and embodiment, *Journal of Aging Studies*, 45(6): 25–31.

Sandhu, S., Lian, T., Connor, D. et al. (2022) Intervention components of link worker social prescribing programmes: A scoping review, *Heath and Social Care in the Community*, 30(6): e3761–e3774. DOI: 10.1111/hsc.14056.

Spracklen, K. (2013) *Leisure, Sports and Society*. Basingstoke: Palgrave Macmillan.

Stebbins, R.A. (1997) Casual leisure: A conceptual statement, *Leisure Studies*, 16(1): 17–25.

World Health Organization (WHO) (2021) *WHO Policy on Disability*. Available at: www.who.int/about/policies/disability (accessed 21 April 2022).

Realm One

The individual, interactions and relationships

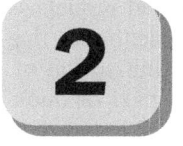

2 Framing meanings of leisure

Sherry D. Dupuis, Colleen Whyte,
Jennifer Carson and Brenda Hounam

Summary

An important aspect of living well for people living with dementia is continued engagement in life. This includes being able to make decisions about your own life. It also involves having access to meaningful activities and caring relationships and being able to continue valued life patterns and routines, such as daily walks around the neighbourhood. Leisure provides an important way for people living with dementia to remain engaged in the world. Yet for people living with dementia, leisure is often seen *only* as therapy. For example, enjoying music and singing becomes music therapy. Enjoying gardening becomes horticultural therapy. This approach is based on professionals' perspectives and denies people living with dementia the opportunity to experience leisure for its own sake. Very little attention has focused on how people living with dementia think about leisure in their own lives. In this chapter, we describe a Canadian project in which we partnered with people living with dementia, family members and professionals to research and understand the meanings of leisure from the point of view of people living with dementia. People living with dementia described how leisure is an important way to celebrate *living*. For example, leisure provides opportunities to be with others, make a difference in the world, grow and develop and have fun. These findings expand our understandings of the meanings of leisure for people living with dementia. They can also help families and professionals to better support people living with dementia in living life to the fullest through leisure.

Introduction

Despite the significance of leisure to the quality of life of people living with dementia in the community and in residential care settings, individuals often lack access to, and are excluded from, opportunities to experience personally valued and meaningful engagements. When available, many approaches to leisure and recreation within the dementia context continue to dismiss the natural value of leisure. In care settings with an emphasis on biomedical models – approaches that make disease, symptom management and physical care the focus – there are increasing institutional pressures towards the 'clinification' of leisure and the arts. Activities and experiences that were once part of one's very essence become therapy (e.g. music therapy, horticultural therapy, pet therapy) used as non-pharmacological interventions with the aim of addressing misunderstood 'behaviours', improving functioning and reducing the 'burden' of care (see for example, Kolanowski et al. 2011; Seitz et al. 2012). While various activity therapies do support specific clinical outcomes, they also objectify and stigmatize people living with dementia when used inappropriately, and they deny opportunities to experience leisure for its own sake.

With the focus on using leisure for medical and functional aims, little attention has been given to how people living with dementia think about leisure in their lives, with most efforts relying on the perspectives of professionals and family. Although including family and professional care partners was an important first step in a (far too long) journey to include the voices of people living with dementia in research and practice, their exclusion continues to be problematic; research demonstrates that staff and family perspectives about what is meaningful to people living with dementia can differ in significant ways from the perspectives of people living with dementia, with staff and family members prioritizing clinical and functional outcomes (Harmer and Orrell 2008). There is a crucial need for more conceptual development on the meanings that people living with dementia themselves attach to leisure to ensure leisure practitioners are better able to support what is most meaningful to them.

To contribute to this conceptual development, the authors of this chapter initiated a large participatory action research project. It was guided by authentic partnerships, an approach that recognizes the capacities of people living with dementia and seeks to work in partnership with diverse stakeholders, including people living with dementia, to challenge stigma and promote inclusion and social justice for all people with dementia (Dupuis et al. 2012a). We brought together a team of people living with dementia, family members, professionals and researchers with the collective aims of:

- opening up possibilities for leisure in the dementia context by prioritizing a conceptualization of leisure grounded firmly in the meanings and experiences of people living with dementia
- supporting the social citizenship of people living with dementia by demonstrating the participatory roles they can play in challenging the status quo.

Our process resulted in the co-creation of the Living and Celebrating Life through Leisure Framework. A detailed description of our participatory process, which included open-ended questionnaires, individual and small group research conversations (some using the arts) with people living with dementia in diverse settings, and photovoice methods, has been published elsewhere (Dupuis et al. 2012b). Integrating our own data and findings with insights from the literature, the primary purpose of this chapter is to present the Framework and to provide examples of how it is being used to better support the leisure lifestyles and well-being of people living with dementia and care partners alike.

The Living and Celebrating Life through Leisure Framework

People living with dementia consistently emphasize how, despite the current focus on servicing the illness, what they really want is to be able to continue to flourish despite dementia. When first diagnosed, 'life is spinning seemingly out of control', like living in the eye of the storm. However, over time 'a rich tapestry of meaningful experiences and understandings [emerge], often facilitated through leisure' (Dupuis et al. 2012b: 246).

From our research, we were able to identify seven common leisure experiences that reflect what people living with dementia need to nurture *living* (see Figure 2.1 below).

Although the leisure experiences are presented separately here, they are highly interconnected, each supporting the others. Different people living with dementia will place more or less importance on each of the experiences at any given moment in time, with some having more or less value or significance at certain times. People with dementia flourish when they have opportunities to engage in all the experiences that are most meaningful to them.

Figure 2.1 The Living and Celebrating Life through Leisure Framework

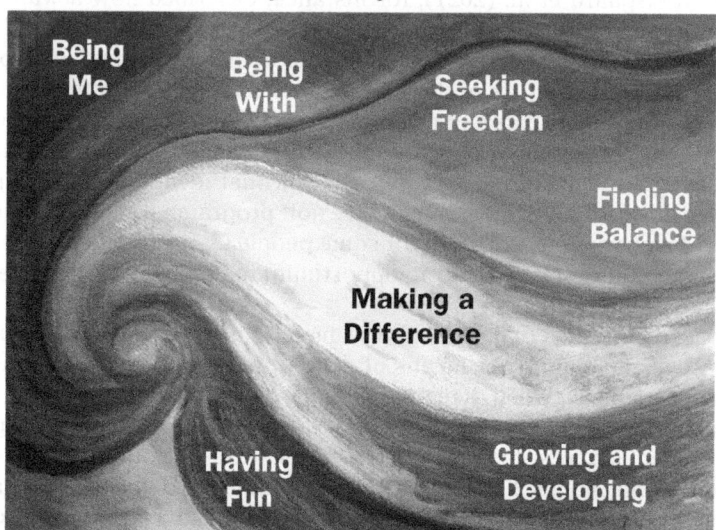

Image created by Dr Lisa Meschino and the members of the John Noble Home LEAD (Leadership, Empowerment, Achievement and Dignity) Program

Being Me

> And the gentleman with the garden, starting with seeds and nurturing it to be something to be enjoyed … and with the carpenters, there again, starting from scratch and being creative … *bringing out your soul*. (Discussion with people living with dementia on meanings of photos connected to *Being Me*)

People living with dementia experience continual threats to their personhood and sense of identity. So it is not surprising that our partners living with dementia describe leisure as a crucial space for *Being Me*, especially when work roles are no longer available to them. *Being Me* recognizes that identity is sustained for people living with dementia and can be expressed in many embodied ways. Consistent with a social citizenship lens, *Being Me* recognizes that our sense of self is not fixed and static, but fluid, evolving over time. It acknowledges the multiple identities and social positions a person living with dementia may occupy, and that they may reveal or conceal different aspects of the self in different contexts depending on the nature of those contexts.

Being Me happens when leisure supports and reaffirms expressions of self and provides opportunities for transformation of self. Other researchers have emphasized the importance of meaningful engagements for maintenance of identity and discovering new aspects of the self (e.g. Han et al. 2016; Górska et al. 2018). In fact, engagements misaligned with valued interests can be detrimental, threatening autonomy and one's sense of self with negative mental health consequences. *Being Me* is supported by past and new activities and often includes experiences that help develop gifts, talents, skills, hobbies and interests.

There are examples of the importance of leisure for *Being Me* in the research literature. Kielsgaard et al. (2021), for instance, described how a walk in the park supported a former postal worker in reconnecting with himself and how a village, specifically designed with people with dementia in mind, supported a woman's valued identity as a shopper. Others have drawn attention to the importance of family rituals and celebrations in supporting the gendered identities and social positions of people living with dementia, and of cultural and spiritual events for nurturing cultural and spiritual identities (Phinney et al. 2013; Han et al. 2016). A dementia-inclusive golf programme supported the construction of a continuous life story for some people living with dementia, while others new to golf described it as an opportunity to create an alternative sense of self (Dupuis et al. 2019).

Arts-based activities (e.g. music, movement, dancing, visual arts) can provide an especially significant means of self-expression for people living with dementia, particularly when they are no longer communicating through words (Han et al. 2016; Wright 2018). Leisure and the arts are also used by people living with dementia to resist stigmatizing identities and to reinforce desired identities (Genoe and Dupuis 2011). While people living with dementia may have to adapt their approaches and expectations about leisure, the meaning attached is not necessarily altered with a diagnosis. For example, one of our partners with dementia describes what *Being Me* means to her:

> Playing the keyboard is something that I do strictly on my own. I use headphones so that no one hears but me and that way I can dream that I play like I used to. I now have to play using sheet music, but every once in a while some tune will come to me, and I feel like it is 20 years ago. It still gives me the most pleasure. I LOVE MY MUSIC.

Through their leisure experiences, people living with dementia demonstrate to themselves and others that they are 'still me' and that they still have worth.

Being With

> If there were a different group of women involved on my dart team, this activity would have gone by the wayside a few years ago. They have done everything possible to keep me involved, even though I don't play nearly as many games as before and I do slow things down. It is the one night out that I have desperately been hanging on to. I actually feel as if I am still part of a team. (Questionnaire response from person living with dementia in the community)

Relational theories place compassionate relationships at the core of human wellness, highlighting that human beings learn, evolve and thrive best in mutual and reciprocal relationships (Jonas-Simpson et al. 2021). People living with dementia often emphasize that they are social beings who still have relational needs and capacity for connection. Despite the importance of relationships to people living with dementia, they are at much higher risks of social isolation and loneliness (Fortune et al. 2021). In fact, a common experience for many people living with dementia is the withdrawal of friends and family who may not know how to communicate and act with them after diagnosis. Couples also report a lack of opportunities to engage in meaningful shared leisure experiences in their communities (Fortune and McKeown 2016). Yet relational efforts of friends and family play a critical role in the continued leisure engagement of people living with dementia (Fortune et al. 2021).

Leisure provides an important space for *Being With*, being with others, where people living with dementia can build and nurture reciprocal, compassionate relationships – feel a part of the world. Thus, leisure experiences that foster a sense of connection and community are highly valued by our partners living with dementia, as this contribution from a person living with dementia shows: '*Being With* means you feel like you belong. You have friends around you, and you belong to something. You're not isolated.'

Researchers have demonstrated how people living with dementia use leisure to make connections with others and how these experiences can nurture relational engagements and communities, particularly when intentionally designed to do so (e.g. Jonas-Simpson et al. 2021; Kielsgaard et al. 2021). For example, music-making spaces can support increased cooperation, interaction and conversation among diverse performers, building cohesion within the group, and providing important opportunities for meaningful engagement *in* community (Dowlen et al. 2018; Tischler et al. 2019; Smith et al. 2022). For others, physical activities such as exercise, golf and dancing provide spaces for social interaction and connection. Wright (2018), for instance, shares the story of Megan who did not communicate with words, but through dance was able to connect in meaningful ways with others. Shared family activities are important for maintaining family relationships and family identity (Phinney et al. 2013). Social clubs such as Memory Boosters, a peer-led social leisure programme for people living with dementia and their care partners (Fortune and McKeown 2016), Leisure Connections, a social recreation group for people with early dementia (Phinney and Moody 2011), and Paul's Club, a social group for people with young-onset dementia (Phinney et al. 2016), create safe spaces for people living with dementia (and care partners) to feel accepted, meet new people, build new friendships and reclaim a place in the community. People with dementia do not just desire connections with people, but also with other meaningful living and non-living things, such as pets, plants and nature (as we discuss under *Seeking Freedom*), valued possessions and higher beings.

Technology, especially during the Covid-19 pandemic, has opened avenues for staying connected, as evidenced by this quote from a project partner living with dementia: 'I have online friends from around the world … Staying in those virtual communities and expanding them has helped me a lot now that I have been forced to retire and move across country to be close to my son.' The intentional creation of social spaces in day programmes (e.g. community support services that provide, for example, an organized programme of activities for people living with dementia and respite for care partners) and residential care settings can support natural and spontaneous connections between residents taking part, family members and professionals, and thus enrich the social environment (Whyte and Fortune 2017).

Being With is also an important space to combat the stigma associated with dementia. Engagement in leisure activities in public spaces, such as art galleries (Camic et al. 2016), or sports grounds through football games (Carone et al. 2016), and dementia-inclusive golf programmes (Dupuis et al. 2019), has potential to create more compassionate communities through raising awareness about dementia and challenging assumptions associated with it. Similarly, Dupuis et al. (2016: 372) demonstrated the possibilities of collaborative arts for personal change and social justice:

> In the community that was created, we all were opened up to the roles and power we have in supporting the citizenship of each other; we all saw new possibilities for actualizing relational citizenship and came to understand how we could do citizenship differently – be better citizens.

The possibilities for challenging the negative stereotypes and misunderstandings of dementia are even more powerful when designed and led by people living with dementia (Dupuis and Gillies 2014).

Seeking Freedom

> It all comes down to being free. (Research conversation with people living with dementia)

Leisure scholar and philosopher, Charles Sylvester (1987: 58) emphasized: 'Leisure … is the celebration of freedom at its crowning point.' This sentiment resonated in our exploration of meanings of leisure for people living with dementia. Living and celebrating life means having opportunities to have a 'break from the norm'. *Seeking Freedom* through leisure provides for this much-needed break, although people living with dementia describe diverse understandings and approaches to *Seeking Freedom*. Some people living with dementia value the spontaneity in life that leisure affords. Others view it as an opportunity to 'escape' the stresses of life and the monotony of day-to-day routines and responsibilities; this can be an important motivation for participation in social leisure programmes (Phinney and Moody 2011; Fortune and McKeown 2016). For some people living with dementia, meaningful leisure experiences provide a necessary escape from their dementia – a way to transcend the disease (Carone et al. 2016). Others describe *Seeking Freedom* as an opportunity to 'get out' of environments that are socially and physically restrictive, such as segregated and locked memory/dementia care units in residential care homes (a description we use with intention); having access to outdoor spaces is important for supporting *Seeking Freedom*. When discussing photographs they had produced reflective of *Seeking Freedom*, one of our partners living with dementia said: 'Obviously nature plays a big part for us; freedom has to do with enjoying nature, whether it be the birds, bees, and blue sky.' In fact, many of the photos shared with us pictured people living with dementia in the outdoors (see Figure 2.2).

Figure 2.2 Examples of photos reflecting Seeking Freedom

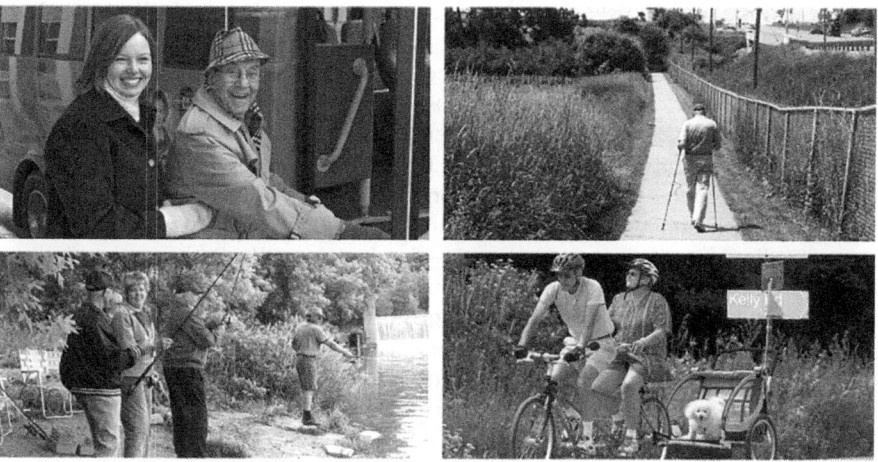

Having access to outdoor spaces was particularly important for our partners living in residential care settings who found life in these settings monotonous and restrictive. One of them describes it in this way: 'It's just the confined … being inside so much. Like you go home, you're inside, you go outside but you're not, again it's freedom. It comes all down to being free.'

Other researchers have noted the importance of access to and use of outdoor spaces as a means of *Seeking Freedom* to re-energize (Olsson et al. 2013) and promote well-being for people living with dementia (Han et al. 2016; Phinney et al. 2016; Górska et al. 2018). In fact, lack of access to outdoor spaces and inadequate support to ensure safe outdoor experiences are associated with loss of freedom, lower levels of self-esteem and psychological well-being and decreased quality of life (Olsson et al. 2013). Given the growing recognition of the importance of *Seeking Freedom* for people living with dementia, Dementia Adventure, a dementia-specific travel programme, was developed in England as a means of providing opportunities for people living with dementia and their families to experience outdoor spaces and a sense of adventure in life (Mapes and Hine 2011).

Seeking Freedom also means having the freedom to make choices and have those choices respected. The intentional construction of freedom in both arts and outdoor spaces can nurture emergent and spontaneous engagement, allow for freedom of movement and support the freedom of choice of people living with dementia (Phinney et al. 2016; Jonas-Simpson et al. 2021). When people living with dementia are excluded from decision-making, including about their leisure lifestyles, and denied access to valued spaces, their social citizenship and quality of life are severely threatened (Bartlett and O'Connor 2010; Birt et al. 2017).

Finding Balance

> I have given up being all things to everyone. I need to pace myself and do what is good for me. (Research conversation with people living with dementia)

Living with dementia has been described as a balancing act, as people living with dementia work to navigate the losses they face with feelings of hope (Genoe and Dupuis 2014). Leisure is essential for *Finding Balance* and, for our partners with dementia, means ensuring balance between relaxation and keeping busy – too much of either is not a good thing.

For people living with dementia who like to be active, *Finding Balance* means finding ways to stay engaged – for instance, through productive or work-related activities or physical activities such as exercise, dancing, going for walks or participating in social programmes. Given the lack of access to meaningful activities, and the barriers and exclusion faced by people living with dementia, it is easy to become bored and withdraw from the world, as one partner with dementia highlights: 'Leisure means to me that I [am] with people to stimulate me and my desire to do challenging things. I have too much time by myself, and I can sometimes become a hermit. I need to be with people, then I feel that I … can still be a productive member of society.' Leisure also provides opportunities to work off accumulated energy built up over days of inactivity, providing a sense of relief and comfort (Wright 2018).

While not having enough meaningful engagements leads to boredom, our partners also emphasize that having too many activities or pressures leads to feeling overwhelmed and stressed. Thus, distractions from the busyness of life, being able to slow down and opportunities for relaxation, solitude and to feel contentment and at peace are also valued. One of our partners describes the connection between *Finding Balance* and leisure like this: '[Leisure] can involve an activity as long as it is simple and relaxing while you enjoy the moment and time you are spending doing it. It can be spent alone or with someone that truly understands my journey. If I am happy and relaxed and not pressured, then I consider that to be leisure.' Another shares how leisure is an important way to regain balance in life when feeling overwhelmed: 'So I can go in and even lay down on the bed and ... turn the radio on and listen to music or the stereo or whatever ... it calms you down that way.' Our partners with dementia use different ways to support this aspect of *Finding Balance*, such as spiritual activities, meditation/reflection, reading, sleeping, sitting in a hot tub, listening to music or watching the television.

The stresses experienced by people living with dementia may increase as the day progresses, causing unnecessary distress, making it particularly important to attend to *Finding Balance* by providing private space and restful and solitary experiences (Han et al. 2016). Also, when people living with dementia take the time to slow down, they are able to 'stop and smell the roses' (Mitchell et al. 2006: 69), see things they haven't noticed before and appreciate the awe and wonder of life around them. When discussing the photos reflecting *Finding Balance*, one of our partners described it like this:

> [It's like] developing yourself in an inner spiritual soul-like way that you didn't take time to do before when you were busy ... Like when you're busy with everyday life, you don't even see the beauty of the weeds and nature ... but when you really look at them, they're beautiful.

Growing and Developing

> Learning that I could learn even with my dementia was so important. (Mitchell et al. 2006: 57)

Because of the stigma associated with dementia it is often assumed that people living with dementia are not able to grow and develop new skills. Yet people living with dementia continue to challenge these misunderstandings. In fact, despite the common push toward so-called 'failure-free activities', not only is maintaining engagement in previously valued pursuits important, people living with dementia also value having opportunities to seek out new challenges and develop new aspects of the self. Leisure provides an important space for *Growing and Developing*.

For some of our partners living with dementia, *Growing and Developing* meant continuing to challenge the mind and body. People living with dementia seek out intellectually and physically stimulating activities – e.g. doing puzzles or exercising – because they perceive these activities as helping them to enhance cognitive and physical abilities and valued skills, improve the ability to perform daily tasks and slow down the progression of the disease (Genoe and Dupuis 2014; Han et al. 2016; Wright 2018).

People living with dementia find meaning in being able to try new activities, take on new roles and learn new knowledge and skills. As examples, our partners with dementia emphasize the importance of their new advocacy roles and supporting research initiatives as co-researchers. Some people living with dementia return to education to finish degrees or learn about new subjects. Participating in cultural and relational arts-based activities, such as through the Culture Bus in the United States and at the Dotsa Bitove Wellness Academy (now The Bitove Method) in Canada, assists all involved in expanding their knowledge about themselves, others and the world (Partners for Livable Communities 2012; Jonas-Simpson et al. 2021). People living with dementia also discover and develop new talents. For instance, one of our partners turned to poetry writing after her diagnosis. Another was enjoying learning a new musical instrument: 'you met Chris today … he's teaching me to play the xylophone … if Chris is here and has free time then we jazz it'. Many people living with dementia learn computer skills so they can feel connected to family, friends and the world, and maintain valued activities in new ways (Cutler et al. 2016).

Growing and Developing through leisure is important for maintaining a sense of hope after diagnosis and promoting meaning in life. In fact, growth may be the strongest predictor of presence of meaning in life for people living with dementia (DeWitte et al. 2021). *Growing and Developing* is also essential for social citizenship as Bartlett and O'Connor (2010: 40) emphasize:

> when talking about the well-being of persons with dementia, it does not make sense to restrict the focus to comfort and a sense of psychological security; it places boundaries on and narrows our understanding of the situation and practices of people with dementia. Moreover, it leaves the field without a structure or language for theorizing the ways in which people with dementia seek to develop, experiment, and grow as citizens.

Further, recognizing and providing opportunities for personal development and to learn new skills challenges the dominant tragedy discourse associated with dementia, enabling positive narratives that defy deficit-focused understandings (Birt et al. 2017).

Making a Difference

> [I would like to] get out and help other people if they'd let me. (Research conversation with people living with dementia)

Leisure provides experiences that fulfil a sense of purpose. For many people living with dementia, this is strongly connected to *Making a Difference* in the world. Our partners with dementia living in the community and in residential care homes desire opportunities to continue to contribute to their own lives, the lives of others, their communities and to the common good. Activities are more meaningful when they provide a sense of feeling valued and offer opportunities to give back. *Making a Difference* through leisure is also an important space to resist dominant assumptions of dementia.

There are many ways that leisure supports experiences of *Making a Difference*. In the following quote, a partner describes how quilting for a new grandchild gave her a new purpose: 'Quilting is always in my hand ... now is another baby coming again so when I make another quilt already for the baby crib.' Others share the pleasure they receive through their dementia advocacy work: 'I am so driven by my newfound purpose to speak up and speak out. I find so much satisfaction from my purposeful activities that I have little time for gardening.' Other researchers have described the active engagement of people living with dementia in raising awareness and campaigning for the rights of people living with dementia (Bartlett 2014). People living with dementia feel a great sense of pride when able to support others and contribute to their communities, as one of our partners explains after being able to help raise money for a new bus: '[The doll house raffle] made a difference in buying a new bus. We raised $400, we did it all by ourselves, and then we presented it to [programme leader].'

Even though *Making a Difference* is extremely meaningful for people living with dementia, they are often not provided with opportunities to do so, perhaps because professionals frequently do not identify this as important for people living with dementia. Yet research highlights the significance *Making a Difference* can have on people living with dementia. For instance, Fortune and McKeown (2016) described how the development of a peer-led social programme addressed the social inequities and exclusion of people living with dementia and their partners in one community by creating a safe space for them to remain engaged *in* community. Moving from a focus on occupation to prioritizing purpose – *Making a Difference* – further supports the social citizenship of people living with dementia.

Having Fun

[During leisure] my heart is at ease and happy when my mind is calm, when my soul feels like singing. (Questionnaire response from person living with dementia in the community)

Central to meanings of leisure for people living with dementia is the experience of *Having Fun*. People with dementia desire opportunities to experience joy, pleasure, enjoyment, happiness, playfulness, mischievousness, and to demonstrate their sense of humour. One partner describes the enjoyment of being able to dance in the middle of the afternoon: 'The [day programme staff] treat you good and of course you dance, people try to anyway ... but at two o'clock in the afternoon! My doctor said heck with this, I'm going there. He says, where else can you go at two in the afternoon and dance?'

Having Fun can happen in diverse ways for people living with dementia. As in other research on experiences of dementia, our partners with dementia emphasize the importance of humour and laughter to *Having Fun* and life quality; humour is an important coping strategy for people living with dementia (Wolverson et al. 2016). One of the dominant experiences of social programmes described by people living with dementia is having fun (Phinney and Moody 2011). In Paul's Club in Canada, for example, walking with others provides an important space for fun (Phinney et al. 2016). Other group activities, such as exercise and dance programmes, collaborative music-making, theatre and relational arts provide opportunities to be humorous, playful and silly and are highly valued by some people living with dementia because of the sense of enjoyment they bring (Wright 2018; Tischler et al. 2019; Jonas-Simpson et al. 2021). Yet because of the focus on clinical and functional outcomes, *Having Fun* is rarely prioritized, as Phinney and Moody (2011: 126) point out:

> Having fun as a feature of group interventions is something that is rarely mentioned in the literature … While improving function, mood, and behaviour may be important program objectives for persons with dementia, living a good life may be a more significant goal, and having the opportunity to laugh and have fun together with other people is vital.

Putting the Framework into practice

Our partners living with dementia felt strongly that the Framework should be shared widely and be accessible to others so it could be used to support people with dementia in living well. One of the ways this was done was through the creation and sharing of a *By Us For Us Guide* focused on the Framework, facilitated by Brenda Hounam and our partners living with dementia (Murray Alzheimer Research and Education Program 2020). We also worked together to create a *Photographic Discussion Guide* using the photos shared by people living with dementia (some of which are included in this chapter) and a set of prompts to be used by professionals as an alternative to traditional assessment approaches and a way of getting to know what is most meaningful to the people living with dementia with whom they work.

In addition, as professionals working in dementia care take up the urgent calls for culture change in dementia and residential care, they are adopting the Framework to shift how they think about and approach leisure and wellness in those settings. As an example, in 2018, Carol Woods Retirement Community in the United States partnered with Jennifer Carson on an initiative called *The Quest Upstream*, with the aim of exploring and documenting the organizational requirements of inclusive living for residents living with dementia, while proactively supporting the well-being of all community members. Central to the project was the belief that the distress people living with dementia might express is not an inherent result of dementia (i.e. so-called 'behaviours') but a sign that aspects of well-being are not being addressed or met. Given its focus on the perspectives of people living with dementia, the team grounded their conceptualization of well-being in the Living and Celebrating Life through Leisure Framework.

Guided by participatory action research, representatives of all members of the Carol Woods community (residents, family care partners and team members) met first in neighbourhood retreats and then regularly in weekly neighbourhood huddles to explore and collaboratively develop an action plan for enabling chosen well-being goals in leisure experiences and activities shaped by our Framework.[1] The process was further supported through daily shift huddles to improve communication, strengthen teamwork and develop and support individual resident well-being plans. The huddles and resident well-being plans are now part of life at Carol Woods. Members of the Carol Woods community believe that the proactive support of well-being guided by the Framework is essential to maintaining their dementia-inclusive approach to care and support.

In another example, the artists at the Dotsa Bitove Wellness Academy (now The Bitove Method), a community arts-based academy grounded in relational caring (Jonas-Simpson et al. 2021) in Canada, used the Framework to guide the focus of relational arts-based engagements with people living with dementia. Using the arts (poetry, visual arts, improvisation, dance, music), people living with dementia, care partners, staff, volunteers and the artists were supported in exploring what the Framework experiences meant for them personally. Every engagement with the Framework provided opportunities for self-discovery and relationship-building for all involved and identified new possibilities for supporting strengths and interests in future programming of activities.

So what does this mean in practice? A call to action

Sylvester (2015: 185) called for 'a critical theory of therapeutic recreation that sustains a posture of re-imagination and change'. The perspectives of people living with dementia, reflected in the Living and Celebrating Life through Leisure Framework, support this call and highlight the need for the liberation of leisure from the therapy culture. We suggest that seeing leisure anew facilitates and nourishes diverse ways of being, being in and relating to the world by both people with dementia and those who support them.

For those supporting or enabling the involvement in leisure of people living with dementia

- Remember that a focus solely on symptom management and clinical and functional outcomes can stigmatize people living with dementia and deny them access to opportunities to have meaningful experiences and flourish.
- Using the Living and Celebrating Life through Leisure Framework ensures that the leisure experiences most meaningful to people living with dementia – *Being Me, Being With, Seeking Freedom, Finding Balance, Growing and*

Developing, Making a Difference and *Having Fun* – are identified, supported and documented.

- Living and Celebrating Life through Leisure must actively include people living with dementia in decision-making about what is most meaningful to them, recognizing that people living with dementia use a range of ways to communicate their experiences and perspectives.
- It is important to regularly revisit the Framework and re-evaluate how perspectives and personal goals might be shifting as people living with dementia continue to change and develop.

For people living with dementia or their informal or family carers

- Think about which of the Living and Celebrating Life through Leisure experiences are most important to the individual concerned – *Being Me, Being With, Seeking Freedom, Finding Balance, Growing and Developing, Making a Difference* and *Having Fun*. Share this information with others and work together to identify ways to support the experiences that are most meaningful.
- Informal or family carers should not assume that they know what is most meaningful to the person living with dementia; they should ask and listen.
- Advocate for the inclusion of people living with dementia in decision-making in research and practice.

Endnote

1 A 'neighbourhood retreat' is a half- to full-day meeting or get-together to which all those living on, working on or visiting a specific floor or unit are invited. In some residential care settings that have embarked on culture change, these floors or units are called 'neighbourhoods'. 'Huddles' are brief meetings held on the floors or other community areas in residential care settings.

References

Bartlett, R. (2014) The emergent modes of dementia activism, *Ageing & Society*, 34(4): 623–44.

Bartlett, R. and O'Connor, D. (2010) *Broadening the Dementia Debate: Towards Social Citizenship*. Bristol: Policy Press.

Birt, L., Poland, F., Csipke, E. and Charlesworth, G. (2017) Shifting dementia discourses from deficit to active citizenship, *Sociology of Health & Illness*, 39(2): 199–211.

Camic, P.M., Baker, E.L. and Tischler, V. (2016) Theorizing how art gallery interventions impact people with dementia and their caregivers, *The Gerontologist*, 56(6): 1033–41.

Carone, L., Tischler, V. and Dening, T. (2016) Football and dementia: A qualitative investigation of a community-based sports group for men with early onset dementia, *Dementia*, 15(6): 1358–76.

Cutler, C., Hicks, B. and Innes, A. (2016) Does digital gaming enable healthy aging for community-dwelling people with dementia?, *Games and Culture*, 11(1–2): 104–29.

Dewitte, L., Vandenbulcke, M., Schellekens, T. and Dezutter, J. (2021) Sources of well-being for older adults with and without dementia in residential care: Relations to presence of meaning and life satisfaction, *Aging and Mental Health*, 25(1): 170–8.

Dowlen, R., Keady, J., Milligan, C. et al. (2018) The personal benefits of musicking for people living with dementia: A thematic synthesis of the qualitative literature, *Arts & Health*, 10(3): 197–212.

Dupuis, S.L. and Gillies, J. (2014) Learning as a vehicle for individual and social transformation: Rethinking leisure education, *Therapeutic Recreation Journal*, 48(2): 113–34.

Dupuis, S.L., Gillies, J., Carson, J. et al. (2012a) Moving beyond patient and client approaches: Mobilizing 'authentic partnerships' in dementia care, support and services, *Dementia*, 11(4): 427–52.

Dupuis, S.L., Kontos, P., Mitchell, G. et al. (2016) Re-claiming citizenship through the arts, *Dementia*, 15(3): 358–80.

Dupuis, S.L., Thompson, K., Middleton, L. and Pearce, B. (2019) Golf-fore-life: Supporting inclusion through dementia-friendly leisure programs. Paper presented at the 48th Annual Scientific and Educational Meeting of the Canadian Association on Gerontology, Moncton, New Brunswick, Canada, October 2019.

Dupuis, S.L., Whyte, C., Carson, J. et al. (2012b) Just dance with me: An authentic partnership approach to understanding leisure in the dementia context, *World Leisure Journal*, 54(3): 240–54.

Fortune, D. and McKeown, J. (2016) Sharing the journey: Exploring a social leisure program for persons with dementia and their spouses, *Leisure Sciences*, 38(4): 373–87.

Fortune, D., Whyte, C. and Genoe, R. (2021) The interplay between leisure, friendship, and dementia, *Dementia*, 20(6): 2041–56.

Genoe, M.R. and Dupuis, S.L. (2011) 'I'm just like I always was': A phenomenological exploration of leisure, identity and dementia, *Leisure/Loisir*, 35(4): 423–52.

Genoe, M.R. and Dupuis, S.L. (2014) The role of leisure within the dementia context, *Dementia*, 13(1): 33–58.

Górska, S., Forsyth, K. and Maciver, D. (2018) Living with dementia: A meta-synthesis of qualitative research on the lived experience, *The Gerontologist*, 58(3): e180–e196.

Han, A., Radel, J., McDowd, J.M. and Sabata, D. (2016) Perspectives of people with dementia about meaningful activities: A synthesis, *American Journal of Alzheimer's Disease & Other Dementias*, 31(2): 115–23.

Harmer, B.J. and Orrell, M. (2008) What is meaningful activity for people with dementia living in care homes? A comparison of the views of older people with dementia, staff and family carers, *Aging and Mental Health*, 12(5): 548–58.

Jonas-Simpson, C., Mitchell, G., Dupuis, S. et al. (2021) Free to be: Experiences of arts-based relational caring in a community living and thriving with dementia, *Dementia*, 21(1): 61–76. DOI: 10.1177/14713012211027016.

Kielsgaard, K., Horghagen, S., Nielsen, D. and Kristensen, H.K. (2021) Moments of meaning: Enacted narratives of occupational engagement within a dementia town, *Journal of Occupational Science*, 28(4): 510–24.

Kolanowski, A., Litaker, M., Buettner, L. et al. (2011) A randomized clinical trial of theory-based activities for the behavioral symptoms of dementia in nursing home residents, *Journal of the American Geriatrics Society*, 59(6): 1032–41.

Mapes, N. and Hine, R. (2011) *Living with Dementia and Connecting with Nature: Exploring the Benefits of Green Exercise with People Living with Dementia*. Colchester: Dementia Adventure.

Mitchell, G.J., Jonas-Simpson, C. and Dupuis, S.L. (2006) *I'm Still Here*. DVD and teaching-learning guide to understanding living with dementia through the medium of the arts. Waterloo, ON: Murray Alzheimer Research and Education.

Murray Alzheimer Research and Education Program (2020) *Living and Celebrating Life through Leisure: An Inspirational Guide for People Living with Dementia*. Series 1. Waterloo, ON: Murray Alzheimer Research and Education. Available at: https://the-ria.ca/resources/by-us-for-us-guides/ (accessed 10 January 2023).

Olsson, A., Lampic, C., Skovdahl, K. and Engström, M. (2013) Persons with early-stage dementia reflect on being outdoors: A repeated interview study, *Aging and Mental Health*, 17(7): 793–800.

Partners for Livable Communities (2012) *Stories for Change: Leadership Examples of Expanding the Arts to New Audiences*. Available at: http://livable.nonprofitsoapbox.com/storage/documents/reports/AIP/Stories_for_Change_final_digital.pdf (accessed 5 October 2021).

Phinney, A., Dahlke, S. and Purves, B. (2013) Shifting patterns of everyday activity in early dementia: Experiences of men and their families, *Journal of Family Nursing*, 19(3): 348–74.

Phinney, A., Kelson, E., Baumbusch, J. et al. (2016) Walking in the neighbourhood: Performing social citizenship in dementia, *Dementia*, 15(3): 381–94.

Phinney, A. and Moody, E.M. (2011) Leisure connections: Benefits and challenges of participating in a social recreation group for people with early dementia, *Activities, Adaptation & Aging*, 35(2): 111–30.

Seitz, D.P., Brisbin, S., Herrmann, N. et al. (2012) Efficacy and feasibility of nonpharmacological interventions for neuropsychiatric symptoms of dementia in long term care: A systematic review, *Journal of the American Medical Directors Association*, 13(6): 503–6.

Smith, S.K., Innes, A. and Bushell, S. (2022) Music-making in the community with people living with dementia and care-partners – 'I'm leaving feeling on top of the world', *Health & Social Care in the Community*, 30(1): 114–23.

Sylvester, C.D. (1987) The politics of leisure, freedom, and poverty, in D. Gold and J. McGill (eds) *The Pursuit of Leisure: Enriching the Lives of People Who Have a Disability*, rev. edn. Downsview, ON: G. Allan Roeher Institute, pp. 57–64. Available at: https://files.eric.ed.gov/fulltext/ED318157.pdf#page=61 (accessed 12 September 2021).

Sylvester, C.D. (2015) Re-imagining and transforming therapeutic recreation: Reaching into Foucault's toolbox, *Leisure/Loisir*, 39(2): 67–191.

Tischler, V., Schneider, J., Morgner, C. et al. (2019) Stronger together: Learning from an interdisciplinary dementia, arts and well-being network (DA&WN), *Arts & Health*, 11(3): 272–7.

Whyte, C. and Fortune, D. (2017) Natural leisure spaces in long-term care homes: Challenging assumptions about successful aging through meaningful living, *Annals of Leisure Research*, 20(1): 7–22.

Wolverson, E.L., Clarke, C. and Moniz-Cook, E.D. (2016) Living positively with dementia: A systematic review and synthesis of the qualitative literature, *Aging and Mental Health*, 20(7): 676–99.

Wright, A. (2018) Exploring the relationship between community-based physical activity and wellbeing in people with dementia: A qualitative study, *Ageing & Society*, 38(3): 522–42.

3 Music in daily life

Becky Dowson

Summary

Throughout our lives, many of us take part in musical activities as a form of leisure. These activities might include listening to recordings, playing an instrument or singing in a choir. For some, music is the focus of their leisure time – their main hobby. For others, music is a more casual interest. Some activities may need training and skill, like playing an instrument. Other activities are open to anyone. In recent years, there has been a lot of interest in musical activities for people living with dementia. Music is thought to have positive effects on mood, memory and quality of life. It can also reduce upsetting symptoms like anxiety, depression and agitation which are more common for people living with dementia. Research has given us evidence of these effects. However, there has been little consideration of music as leisure for people living with dementia. This may be because many people will still think of the person with dementia as a patient – someone who is ill – and of music as a treatment for the dementia. Instead, people living with dementia should be seen as citizens who may use music in their leisure time, like anyone else. In this chapter we look at the example of a singing group for people living with dementia and their care partners to see why singing group members joined the group and what they got from it. Understanding this could be helpful to empower people living with dementia to take part in musical leisure in whatever way they choose.

Introduction

People engage with music as a leisure activity in many different ways over the course of their lives. Some of these activities involve no skill or training; others require expertise or musical equipment. Even for people who do not have any particular interest in music, it is likely that music will nevertheless have a place in their leisure time. However, motivation to seek out and engage with music, and the kinds of activities which are sought, vary widely from person to person.

The aim of this chapter is to look at the role of music as a leisure activity in the lives of people living with dementia. There is growing research evidence that music can have beneficial effects for people living with dementia, such as improving mood and reducing neuropsychiatric symptoms (non-cognitive symptoms related to dementia, such as anxiety or depression), leading to enhanced well-being. This focus has led to music being seen in many circles as a treatment for dementia and its symptoms. Consequently, it appears that the idea of music as a leisure activity for people with dementia has been somewhat neglected.

This chapter will first consider the many forms that musical leisure may take in the context of Stebbins' (1997) concepts of serious and casual leisure. We will look at some of the existing literature about musical leisure and dementia. We will then examine how the focus on music as a 'treatment' for dementia has affected attitudes to music as leisure for people living with the condition, and explore whether music does have special properties relevant to people living with dementia. The example of a real singing group will then be used to explore the motivations of people living with dementia for taking part in musical activities. The author played a leading role in the UK research that accompanied this initiative, some of the findings of which are set out later. To conclude, we will think about how people living with dementia can be empowered to take part (or not) in musical leisure in whatever way they choose.

Music in daily life

When we think about what music means to us in our daily lives, we will all have different ideas and associations. Some of us are professional musicians, but for most of us music is something we do in our leisure time. The kinds of musical leisure we engage with depend not only on our preferences, shaped by our culture and upbringing, but also on our skills, free time, opportunities, financial resources and our perceptions of our own musicality. Similar-sounding activities may involve very different levels of skill and investment of time and energy. For example, think of someone who says 'I sing in a choir'. For one person, this activity may involve irregular attendance at a weekly singing session which is open to anyone and requires no musical training. For another, it may mean the intensive programme of individual practice, rehearsals and concerts which come with singing in an accomplished amateur choir. Even more passive activities, such as listening to music, will be experienced differently depending on the listener's background and knowledge.

Stebbins has proposed the idea of serious and casual leisure as a framework for understanding the ways that humans spend their leisure time. In his formulation, serious leisure is 'the systematic pursuit of an amateur, a hobbyist, or a volunteer activity sufficiently substantial and interesting for the participant to find a career there in the acquisition and expression of a combination of its special skills, knowledge, and experience' (Stebbins 1997: 17). The use of the term 'career' is significant, implying a journey of skill acquisition with defined progression. Casual leisure is then defined by Stebbins as any leisure activity outside the definition of serious leisure as 'immediately, intrinsically rewarding, relatively short-lived pleasurable activity requiring little or no special training to enjoy it' (Stebbins 1997: 18). Considering music, it is straightforward to think of clear examples of serious leisure (e.g. lifelong study and mastery of an instrument) versus casual leisure (e.g. turning on the radio while you're doing the dishes). However, an activity which appears the same for everyone, such as attending a concert, could be experienced as a form of casual leisure by some and as serious leisure by others.

People's engagement with music is affected by their sense of their own musicality. It is not uncommon to hear someone claim that they are 'unmusical' or 'tone-deaf'. These people sometimes consider themselves unworthy of participation in active music-making because of a perceived lack of ability (Ruddock and Leong 2005). Negative comments about a person's musicality made early in life can become deeply embedded in their sense of musical identity and remain influential for years. I have met people who were told off by teachers for singing out of tune, or called tone-deaf; decades later, these comments still deter people from taking part in activities they might enjoy. True deficits in musical perception (e.g. congenital amusia) are uncommon, and research has suggested that many people who self-describe as tone-deaf do not have any perceptual difficulties (Cuddy et al. 2005). However, there has been a belief in Western society that musicality is an innate gift granted to a select few, and that active music-making should be left to these experts. This assumption has been challenged in music psychology research by the theory that musicality is a normal facet of cognitive development in a musical environment (Serafine 1988). Meanwhile, Trevarthen (2008) proposes that the vocal interactions between babies and their caregivers are rooted in a 'communicative musicality' which precedes the development of language in all humans.

People living with dementia – patients or citizens?

In the last two decades, much research has focused on the potential benefits of music for people living with dementia, reflected by increased awareness and provision of musical activities specifically for them. For example, in the United Kingdom groups such as Singing for the Brain (community singing sessions aimed at people living with dementia and their carers, run by the Alzheimer's Society) have become popular and widespread. The National Institute for Health and Care Excellence also now includes a recommendation of music therapy in its quality standard for people living with dementia (NICE 2019).

Evidence suggests that music may decrease symptoms such as agitation, anxiety and depression and improve cognition among people living with dementia (Särkämö et al. 2014; van Der Steen et al. 2018). These effects in turn can improve quality of life, decrease prescription of antipsychotic medication and delay the need for residential care, thus reducing demand on health and social care services. As music is non-invasive, relatively cheap and has benefits for people living with dementia, its appeal to researchers, healthcare professionals and policymakers is understandable. The potential of music in this area is real and exciting, and this chapter is not intended to downplay these important advances.

However, in the way music for people living with dementia tends to be characterized, and in the language used to describe its potential benefits, music is often portrayed as a treatment for dementia rather than a leisure activity. People living with dementia are viewed as patients, and music is the 'drug' which is prescribed to treat their condition. Consider this passage from the Cochrane review of music-based interventions for people living with dementia:

> Dementia is a clinical syndrome with a number of different causes which is characterized by deterioration in cognitive, behavioural, social and emotional functions. Pharmacological interventions are available but have limited effect to treat many of the syndrome's features. Less research has been directed towards non-pharmacological treatments. (van der Steen et al. 2018: 1)

The text focuses exclusively on the syndrome and its treatments, neglecting to mention the people who are living with it. Kitwood's concepts of personhood and person-centred care (Kitwood 1997), and more recent ideas of social citizenship have helped to move the focus of dementia care away from this biomedical model (Bartlett and O'Connor 2007). Treating people living with dementia as patients with respect to their access to music could be seen as a form of discrimination against this group of citizens on the basis of a medical condition, and ignores the role that music may have played as a leisure activity throughout their lives.

Music as treatment or music as leisure

So far, this chapter has discussed how most of us engage in serious or casual musical leisure. Our self-perception as musical or unmusical influences the degree to which we engage with music. Music can be a complex part of our social and cultural identity. We have also seen how a growing interest in musical activities for people living with dementia has been coupled with a tendency to view such activities as a treatment for dementia, rather than a leisure activity. The therapeutic potential of music for people living with dementia should not be ignored. However, as we have seen, there are some problems with this 'music as treatment' paradigm:

1 It portrays people living with dementia as patients in need of treatment rather than citizens with as much right to take part in musical leisure (or not) as anyone else.
2 It means that if a musical activity 'doesn't work' (is not effective in reducing dementia-related symptoms) it may be dismissed, when it actually has real value in other ways. Healthcare research funders and commissioners may reject proposals unless they can show symptom reduction.
3 It undermines the perspective of the person living with dementia by prioritizing *objective* symptom reduction over *subjective* experience of the activity.
4 It risks tailoring activities to the condition rather than the person, assuming that because someone has a dementia diagnosis, music will be an appropriate activity for them.

The role of music specifically as a leisure activity for people living with dementia is therefore an important but neglected area. Sixsmith and Gibson (2007) state that although the therapeutic benefits of music have been explored, little has been written about music in the everyday lives of people living with dementia. Their qualitative research illuminates the 'fundamental and multifaceted role' of music in everyday life, finding that most people 'enjoyed music as an activity in and of itself through their emotional responses to the music' (Sixsmith and Gibson 2007: 132). Music was seen as promoting involvement and engagement in everyday activities; for some, it was 'an active, enriching and embedded part of their everyday lives and it enhanced their sense of well-being' (Sixsmith and Gibson 2007: 132).

However, participants in this research identified problems too: some found it hard to articulate their preferences about music, and several had hearing impairments which interfered with their access to music. For others, their dementia affected their confidence about taking part in activities. For example, one man living with dementia in the study, Robert, had been a regular stage performer, but now doubted his ability to perform: 'Oh I could sing, but I'd be worried I'd forget the words, forget what I was singing, I'd look a fool. No, I'd like to do it, but I just don't think I could anymore' (Sixsmith and Gibson 2007: 138). For people who have been heavily involved with music, Robert's words illustrate that cognitive impairment can bring a real or perceived sense of loss of skill, and a mourning for these abilities which may complicate their future relationship with music and discourage them from taking part in activities they once enjoyed.

The power of music?

It is common to encounter the suggestion that music has a special power for people living with dementia, that music can reignite the memory and stimulate in a way that may appear transformative. This property of music is relevant to music as leisure because it says something about the accessibility of the medium. If the particular attributes of music mean that it remains accessible and meaningful throughout the progression of a person's dementia, it may gain increasing relevance as a leisure activity for them, especially if other forms of leisure become less relevant and music is able to fill their place. Although we do not necessarily expect someone's preferences to change with the onset of dementia, they may shift if former activities become more difficult and/or less meaningful. This could lead to music becoming a very important part of the life of a person living with dementia, when previously they would not have favoured it over other leisure activities. It is also possible (though anecdotally it seems less common) for a person living with dementia to find that music is less meaningful, or that their preferences have radically changed.

McDermott, Orrell and Ridder (2014) conducted a qualitative study to understand the importance of music for people living with dementia, and used their findings to develop a psychosocial model of music in dementia which 'goes beyond the idea of music as a tool to fix a behavioural problem (e.g. agitation) suggesting that it is part of a wider appreciation of life' (McDermott, Orrell and Ridder 2014:

713). The model centres around three interconnected properties of music: 'Who you are' (cultural and personal identity), 'Here and now' (music stimulates immediate, in the moment responses) and 'Connectedness' (music is a vehicle for shared interaction). The authors point out that the findings of their study have many similarities with research conducted in Australia by Hays and Minichiello (2005) with a sample of older adults (it is not specified whether any of them had a cognitive impairment, but all lived independently). The Australian study found that music helped protect people's sense of identity, fostered social connections and reduced isolation, and provided an experience of spirituality. The similarities suggest that the meaningfulness of music for older people is shared by people living with and without dementia.

In the next section, we will use the example of a singing group for people living with dementia and their carers to investigate the role that this musical activity played in the attendees' lives, their experience of the group and their motivations for taking part.

Case example: The singing group

The group in question was set up as part of a research study in which I was involved. It took place in the communal area of a sheltered housing[1] complex and was open both to residents and external attendees. When recruiting for the study, we included people living with dementia or memory problems, and their carers or supporters. We did not want to exclude people with mild cognitive impairment, or those who might be experiencing the early signs of dementia but had yet to seek a diagnosis, as it was felt the group could be particularly helpful for people at this stage. The participants were invited to attend ten weekly singing sessions.

The singing group sessions took place in the morning, lasted about an hour and were followed by refreshments. The sessions were led by a facilitator with no prior experience of leading activities of this kind using a manual designed as a guide for novice facilitators (evaluating the manual was one aim of the study). After a warm-up, the group sang a selection of songs from a songbook specially created for the sessions. Group members had the chance to choose what songs to sing, and to suggest songs for future sessions. During the sessions, I played the piano for the group.

Participants were interviewed before they started coming to the singing group, and after they had attended ten sessions. Two focus groups were also held towards the end of the course of sessions. All the interviews and focus groups were audio or video recorded, and the recordings transcribed and anonymized prior to analysis. Since participants were interviewed before and after the sessions, insight was gained into their motivations for attending the singing group, their feelings about their own musicality, as well as their experience of the sessions themselves and any changes in their lives that had resulted from them. The following sections describe some of these findings, using the participants' own words as much as possible. The findings are reported selectively, focusing on those most relevant to the present topic of music as leisure. It should be noted that judgements about musicality and singing ability all came from the participants themselves, and do not reflect any opinion about the participants' musical abilities on my part.

Musical experience and sense of musical self

For some participants it was clear that music had consistently been a very important part of their life. 'The house has always been full of music' commented one person living with dementia, while another said 'Music's really been one of the main things in my life. I wouldn't give it up unless I really had to.' These people had often been involved in playing instruments or singing, sometimes to a semi-professional standard. For others, music was a significant part of their lives, but they were involved in less active types of music-making. One carer said to her husband, who was living with dementia: 'You like coming in here and putting your headphones on or just – just listening, don't you?' Two people said that music had not really been particularly important to them.

Some group members implied they had some musical skill, although it seemed that modesty prevented them from stating this explicitly. On the other hand, several participants said that they considered themselves bad at singing; one person living with dementia commented 'I can't sing, but I just enjoy it', while another group member living with memory problems said 'I've got a terrible voice so I would never present myself at any sort of a choir.'

Several of the group members were current or former participants in organized singing activities. Three sang in different local choirs, while others attended a casual singing group. One had recently given up singing in a choir, in her words 'because I've got dementia'. Even though she had loved being in the choir, she felt that she would not have been able to keep up.

People with a range of musical backgrounds put themselves forward to take part in the group. For some, active music-making had already played a significant role in their lives, and they may have considered music a form of serious leisure. For others, this might have been the first time since childhood that they had taken part in group singing, and music was a more casual leisure pursuit.

Motivations for joining the group

Many people said that their main reason for taking part in the study was that they found singing enjoyable or hoped they would enjoy it. This comment from a person living with memory problems was typical: 'I have really no expectations at all, other than I think I would enjoy it.' One couple mentioned that they appreciated the chance to 'try something new'. Others thought that the group would provide pleasurable anticipation, as well as simply 'something to do', as one person with dementia remarked.

For some, the specific benefits of singing were a motivation for taking part. One couple had read that singing could be good for you 'whether you can sing or not'. Several people believed singing could have cognitive benefits. One person with memory problems felt that singing could keep one's brain active: 'I think you keep your brain going, if you're singing, your brain's working.' A carer whose husband was living with dementia and was an experienced choral singer felt it was important for him to keep singing as he was still able to remember the words to songs, even though his use of speech was declining.

Many participants were motivated by the potential opportunity for meeting new people, finding company and rekindling a social life which might have become more limited in recent years. One carer said that she wanted her mum 'to go out a bit more and socialise 'cos she always used to be a social sort of person'.

The singing group attracted a range of people with diverse motivations for attending. Many of these reasons were nothing particularly to do with dementia and could equally apply to any person at a similar stage of life, such as looking for an enjoyable activity to pass the time or wishing to meet people and make friends. For others, it was the specific benefits of singing for people living with dementia which spoke to them. And many had a mixture of reasons for choosing to come to the group, recognizing the potential for the singing group to have diverse social and psychological benefits.

Experiences of the sessions

Most participants who completed the interview and focus groups after the sessions were positive about the group. Some used superlative language when talking about their feelings, saying that they had loved the sessions, that they were 'marvellous' or the 'highlight of the week'. Others said that they liked the group and had enjoyed it. Only one person said that she was not impressed with the sessions, although she was unable to say exactly why. The group members said that they found the session atmosphere to be relaxed and happy, with a sense of fun. Most participants felt that the group had evolved over time as everyone got to know each other, and this had made people more relaxed and comfortable about trying new things.

Many participants appreciated the sense that the group was about the enjoyment of singing rather than being good at it, and that it was OK to make mistakes. This ethos was promoted and modelled by the group facilitator, herself not a professional musician. The result was that the group members who were not experienced singers felt reassured and safe in participating. One person with dementia felt that 'you don't have to be a proper singer', while a carer liked the group because it was 'very relaxed, it's not you've got to sing in tune'. The group provided a space for active making which appeared to feel safe and permissive for most of the group members, including those without previous singing experience or who thought of themselves as unmusical or non-singers.

Benefits or changes in everyday life

Several participants found the experience of singing enjoyable or uplifting. 'You can't be sad if you're singing' said one person with dementia, while a carer used the evocative phrase, 'it dusted a few feathers off me again, and it brought the spark back'. For some people, these qualities of singing were experienced during the singing itself, and for others they carried over into a longer-lasting change in mood, like the person living with memory problems who said, 'I came away feeling uplifted.'

Attending the group gave routine to some participants' weeks. Many looked forward to the sessions, and one used the phrase 'keeping things going' to describe how she felt the sessions motivated her. Another group member said that she enjoyed the sessions because 'it was not me doing nothing'. The sessions also seemed to have an effect on the musical lives of some participants. Two people who had described themselves as unable to sing felt more confident about using their voices; one was even thinking of joining a community choir. Furthermore, one couple said they were now singing at home together.

Benefits to memory and cognition were widely reported by the group members. For example, one carer described how her mother was simultaneously using several different cognitive skills when she took part in the sessions, such as reading the lyrics and remembering the tune. She felt this had helped to improve her mother's concentration. Participants felt that singing well-known songs could 'ignite' their memories. Several people described how being able to remember songs and lyrics was a positive experience for them, such as this person living with dementia who said: 'I can, you know, remember a lot of it, a lot of what's there, now that we've been doing it, and it seems to – it sticks, that's the big thing.' Singing these familiar songs seemed to stimulate recall spontaneously and without effort.

Finally, the opportunity for social interaction and support was widely reported by the group members as a benefit. The group provided a chance to make new friends, as one carer described: 'As time's gone on everybody's sort of got more integrated and everybody seems to get on very well together.' Another carer commented: 'I do wonder sometimes if half of them go for the biscuits or the singing, you know.' Although humorous, this comment suggests that for some the social time spent over refreshments may be more important than the singing.

The group was also a chance for people with shared experience of dementia and memory problems to be together in a supportive atmosphere. The sessions did not focus on dementia; it was enough that the participants understood their mutual reason for being there. One person living with dementia described her sense of 'that kind of feeling that you're there with a group of people who are in a similar position'. Carers and people living with dementia also found practical advice and emotional support from other members. As one carer put it, 'It's a support network, which is a real added bonus.'

Overall, the group members reported various benefits from attending the sessions. Some found the group gave them something to do and to look forward to, as well as bringing routine to their week. The act of singing was frequently found to be enjoyable and uplifting, resulting in short-term effects on mood, some of which may have been longer lasting. Some people said that taking part in the sessions motivated them to try other music activities outside the group.

The group members also found support and friendship with people in a similar situation, resulting in practical and emotional benefits. Some of these benefits might be characterized as 'leisure', such as simple enjoyment and the opportunity to meet people. Others with specific relevance to dementia are more similar to 'treatment', such as the stimulation of memory and cognition. However, it is important to consider the benefits of such activities in terms of what people living with dementia think is meaningful, rather than exclusively what researchers or clinicians have decided is important.

Experienced musicians in the group

The singing group included several people with a lot of musical experience. This is given a particular focus because it gives insight into the complex ways that musical expertise may affect participation in leisure activities, both positively and negatively. One pair who took part in the study had extensive choral experience and considered that music had played a big part in their lives. However, from the outset they were concerned that their experience would mark them out as different in the group and might make others feel self-conscious. In fact, this dyad dropped out of the study after attending the first three sessions. Their reason for leaving was that the kind of singing that the group was doing was not at a level which suited them.

Another person living with dementia who attended the group was an experienced instrumental player. She completed the course of sessions, but her feedback was not positive, commenting 'I'm not terribly impressed by what you're doing, which isn't very complimentary I'm afraid.' We discussed her previous musical experience and she said 'I'm a bit critical', implying that perhaps the sessions did not meet the standards of music-making to which she was used.

On the other hand, one of the group members had been a prolific singer in amateur stage productions. She had given this up a few years previously because of age-related changes in her voice. However, after attending the group for several weeks, she sang a solo to the rest of the group and commented 'to have the opportunity to sing, it works wonders for me'. Afterwards, she said that she no longer noticed the changes in her voice.

The experiences of these musicians show the difficulty of pitching a session so that it accommodates diverse desires, skills and preferences. We tried to be as inclusive as possible, but it may not be feasible to run a group which suits absolutely everyone. Although this was not universally the case, in our singing group it appears that the more musically experienced participants were more likely to find it less suited to their needs. In general, it may be that people used to engaging with music as a serious leisure activity may find it difficult to switch to a more casual way of relating to music as leisure, such as an inclusive singing group.

Maintaining and facilitating participation

Bearing in mind the diversity in people's cultural heritage, musical experiences, personal preferences and current abilities, this section brings together the principles discussed throughout the chapter and presents a way of putting them into practice. Informed by the case study, the questions below are intended to start conversations about how people living with dementia can be empowered to take part in musical leisure activities in whatever way suits them best. They may also be helpful to determine what kinds of music experience would be most appropriate for an individual. These questions are aimed at people living with dementia and their family and professional carers.

1 What musical leisure activities did the person living with dementia take part in prior to their diagnosis?
2 Is there any reason why this person cannot continue with their previous activities now?
3 If the answer to 2 is 'yes', what could be done to modify or tailor the activities so they can continue to take part?
4 If they cannot continue with their previous activities, is there a similar activity they could join or take part in?
5 If the person living with dementia is an expert musician, what support do they need to sustain their expertise post-diagnosis?
6 If the person living with dementia did not previously have many musical leisure activities, is there a particular reason to think their engagement with music may be different now?
7 What information about a person's life history, preferences, tastes and culture can be used to inform what musical leisure activities are offered?

The following fictional vignette shows how some of these principles might play out in practice. Understanding how needs change over time is important in determining choice of musical activity.

Vignette: Mrs G

Mrs G had always enjoyed singing in the choral society and performing in their concerts. She continued to sing with them following her dementia diagnosis, but after a while she began to find it difficult to follow the pace of the rehearsals and find her place in the music. From then on, Mrs G's friend always sat next to her to help her if needed. This worked well for a while, but Mrs G was having increasing difficulty reading the notes, making it hard for her to learn new pieces. Reluctantly, she decided she would have to give up singing in the choral society. However, she started attending a local community singing group instead, with her daughter. This group did not use musical scores, so it suited Mrs G, although the music chosen was usually pop music from the 1960s and 70s which Mrs G didn't like as much as classical music. However, Mrs G enjoys listening to this kind of music on her CDs at home, and at the choral society concerts which she still attends.

Concluding thoughts

This chapter has discussed music in the daily lives of people living with dementia. We saw at the beginning of the chapter that our response to music is mediated by our sense of our own musicality, skills and training and previous experiences with music. Music has been singled out as a powerful medium for improving the lives of people living with dementia, but in harnessing its power we should not prioritize someone's diagnosis of dementia over their preferences, personality and previous experiences. Music is accessible for many people living with dementia, and importantly it often remains meaningful and comprehensible throughout the progression of the illness. However, we should avoid assuming that, because someone has a diagnosis of dementia, they will automatically appreciate and engage with music. It may be especially complicated for people who are 'serious leisure' musicians, who may not find inclusive, general musical events suitable for their tastes, and may mourn the loss of previous skills. A person-centred view of music for people living with dementia will prioritize the preferences and previous experiences of the individual above their diagnosis and will avoid viewing music purely as a treatment for dementia.

So what does this mean in practice?

For those supporting or enabling the involvement in leisure of people living with dementia

- People's use of music as a leisure activity is shaped by their personal history, experiences, culture and identity.
- People living with dementia should be supported to continue with their existing musical leisure activities.
- If this is not possible, suitable similar alternatives should be found.

For people living with dementia or their informal or family carers

- Music is a valuable leisure activity for many people living with dementia.
- There is no reason to assume someone's musical preferences will change after diagnosis.
- Expert musicians living with dementia may find it difficult to adjust to changes in their skill and proficiency.

For researchers

- Music shows promise as a non-pharmacological treatment for some dementia symptoms, but this should not eclipse its value as a leisure activity.
- Understanding the value of music in everyday life for people living with dementia is a promising topic for future research.

Acknowledgements

Many thanks to Dr Ruby Swift for her help in developing the early plans for this chapter.

Endnote

1 'Sheltered housing' in the UK describes a housing complex for older or disabled people. Residents live independently in private units with some shared facilities, and a manager or warden has oversight.

References

Bartlett, R. and O'Connor, D. (2007) From personhood to citizenship: Broadening the lens for dementia practice and research, *Journal of Aging Studies*, 21(2): 107–18.

Cuddy, L.L., Balkwill, L.L., Peretz, I. and Holden, R.R. (2005) Musical difficulties are rare: A study of 'tone deafness' among university students, *Annals of the New York Academy of Sciences*, 1060(1): 311–24.

Hays, T. and Minichiello, V. (2005) The contribution of music to quality of life in older people: An Australian qualitative study, *Ageing and Society*, 25(2): 261–78.

Kitwood, T. (1997) *Dementia Reconsidered: The Person Comes First*. Maidenhead: Open University Press.

McDermott, O., Orrell, M. and Ridder, H.M. (2014) The importance of music for people with dementia: The perspectives of people with dementia, family carers, staff and music therapists, *Aging & Mental Health*, 18(6): 706–16.

NICE (2019) *Dementia Quality Standard* (QS184). Available at https://www.nice.org.uk/guidance/qs184 (accessed 25 May 2022).

Ruddock, E. and Leong, S. (2005) 'I am unmusical!': The verdict of self-judgement, *International Journal of Music Education*, 23(1): 9–22.

Särkämö, T., Tervaniemi, M., Laitinen, S. et al. (2014) Cognitive, emotional, and social benefits of regular musical activities in early dementia: Randomized controlled study, *The Gerontologist*, 54(4): 634–50.

Serafine, M.L. (1988) *Music as Cognition: The Development of Thought in Sound*. New York: Columbia University Press. Available at: https://books.google.com/books/about/Music_as_Cognition.html?id=uOc7lIjLu2wC (accessed 27 October 2021).

Sixsmith, A. and Gibson, G. (2007) Music and the wellbeing of people with dementia, *Ageing & Society*, 27(1): 127–45.

Stebbins, R.A. (1997) Casual leisure: A conceptual statement, *Leisure Studies*, 16(1): 17–25.

Trevarthen, C. (2008) The musical art of infant conversation: Narrating in the time of sympathetic experience, without rational interpretation, before words, *Musicae Scientiae*, (special issue): 15–46.

van der Steen, J.T., van Soest-Poortvliet, M.C., van der Wouden, J.C. et al. (2018) Music-based therapeutic interventions for people with dementia (Review), *Cochrane Database of Systematic Reviews*, 5(5): 1–86.

4 Gender, leisure and dementia

Rebecca Oatley

Summary

This chapter looks at how gender can shape leisure experiences. Gender is the sense of what it means to be a man, a woman or non-binary. Gender effects how we act and interact. It can influence what actions and attributes we expect of different people. Expectations of gender can shape how we interpret leisure activities. Rigid gender stereotypes can mean certain leisure activities privilege some people over others. For example, boxing is often associated with men, netball with women. This chapter uses examples from my study of women's experiences of sport reminiscence in the UK to demonstrate how gender can shape leisure opportunities. Many women experience meaningful connections to sport, and yet sport reminiscence activities are often centred on traditional ideas linking men to sport. The language and behaviour of individuals and groups can reinforce stereotypes, which can be unhelpful to people whose identities vary from such rigid ideas. This can prevent people from accessing or being offered leisure opportunities they might enjoy and that can help them experience playing an active role in everyday life. Examples offered in the chapter also demonstrate that sport as leisure (both as activity and topic of conversation) can be a valuable context in which gender-based stereotypes are challenged. Taking part in leisure can offer people the opportunity to experience gender in ways that feel well-aligned with their sense of self. This can only happen if people are offered choice and control over their preferred leisure activities and practitioners are aware of the impact gender-based assumptions might have on different people.

Introduction

Gender can shape leisure experiences for people living with dementia. Gendered identity is a person's internal experience of what it means to be a man, a woman or non-binary (a term for people whose gender identity doesn't sit comfortably with man or woman). A sense of gender can be an important aspect of identity and what it means to feel like a human being. Leisure can be a means through which gendered identities are upheld. The limited research base connecting dementia and gender is considered, and the problem with binary gender constructions is introduced. The chapter then turns to a recent study of sport reminiscence I conducted, which helps to demonstrate ways in which gender can affect leisure opportunities for people living with dementia.

Gender is a social construct (a shared idea that has been created by society) that shapes life experiences. For example, traditional constructions of gender associate strength and power with being male, whereas grace and beauty are more commonly associated with being female. Gender should not be confused with biological sex and should not be considered a binary divide between men and women. The concept of gender is fluid, and constructions are developed through our life experiences, social culture and relationships. Gender is relational, which means that roles do not exist in isolation, but are defined in relation to other people. Thus, gendered assumptions can create inequality and power hierarchies between people.

The social construction of gender can influence the ways in which we act and are expected to act. Given how gender can affect life experiences, it is perhaps a surprise that it has largely been overlooked in dementia care policy and practice. We know that how people are treated influences their experience of dementia, and yet we rarely consider how gender might shape interactions.

Gender, leisure and dementia

Leisure is a broad topic that includes a wide range of activities. Some leisure activities have strong gendered connotations within different cultures. For example, in the United Kingdom, football (soccer) is often associated with men, whereas knitting is typically assumed to be a female leisure activity. These are not examples of biological difference; rather, they are gender-based assumptions that have been constructed by the culture in which they exist. When a leisure activity is closely aligned to assumptions, it can make it an exclusive location where only certain people with particular identities are accepted.

Leisure can be life-enhancing and can support people and their families to live well with dementia. Leisure opportunities can enable people to experience enjoyment and pleasure, reinforce a sense of unique identity, feel a sense of belonging and place in the world and resist common stigma associated with dementia. However, people living with dementia can feel a loss of identity because of their symptoms and the way in which the world responds to them. Loss of gendered identity can be a part of this. Participation in leisure activities can offer opportunities to (re)experience a sense of gendered identity that might otherwise be lost because of symptoms of dementia or older age. However, leisure activities can also be associated with gender-based stereotyping. A person's sense of gendered identity does not necessarily emulate gender stereotypes. As researchers, practitioners and people affected by dementia, it is important to note that certain activities can be assumed more appropriate for certain genders. For people who affiliate their identity with this set of assumptions, the activity might be valuable; however, other people might find assumptions create barriers that make it difficult to access activities they might enjoy. This can undermine the person's identity and sense of place in the world. In this book, leisure is framed through the lens of social citizenship. This means that opportunities to take part in leisure, and access the potential outcomes that it provides, are viewed as a right for people living with dementia. In turn, this means that greater attention to the complex point at which gender, dementia and leisure meet must be considered if we are to best uphold opportunities for citizenship for people living with dementia.

Gender-centric leisure

One area where gender has begun to feature in the dementia care field is in the development of male-centric leisure activities. This has been a response to the observation that men can be reticent to get involved in group social activities (Clark et al. 2015). It has been suggested that activities may be perceived as too feminine, or because men find themselves at a numerical disadvantage in groups for older people (Gleibs et al. 2011). In recent years, leisure activities have been developed that are intended to appeal specifically to men, such as sport-based activity, sport reminiscence, Men's Sheds, allotment work and men's clubs (e.g. Schofield and Tolson 2010; Gleibs et al. 2011; Carone et al. 2014; Anstiss et al. 2018).

Sport has long been underpinned by a masculine hegemony that reinforces particular ideas of masculinity. Of course, sport is a diverse topic that includes many activities with different gender-based assumptions. However, sports-based activities for people living with dementia have largely focused on a common belief that there is a natural connection between men and sport. This assumption is linked to idealized masculine traits, such as power and strength.

Men's Sheds is a gendered leisure activity reported to be successful in Australia, the UK and in the Republic of Ireland. It involves a focus on manual skill, woodwork and practical activities for groups of older men, including those living with dementia (see Anstiss et al. 2018). As with sport-based activities, Men's Sheds is based on traditional ideas of what 'being a man' entails.

Research has suggested that Men's Sheds and sport-based activities can offer valuable opportunities for men to demonstrate and experience a sense of gender, gendered relations and gendered ideals that might otherwise feel lost in the wider context of living with dementia (Schofield and Tolson 2010; Carone et al. 2014; Anstiss et al. 2018). In a study of football-based physical activity for men living with young onset dementia, staff suggested that the all-male dynamic of group activity was particularly beneficial as it replicated a masculine working environment (Carone et al. 2014). A similar finding was noted with respect to Men's Sheds (Anstiss et al. 2018). However, recent research in football reminiscence noted that some men preferred groups where women were present and where this presence tempered the hypermasculine culture that might otherwise dominate (Sass et al. 2021). This demonstrates that gendered environments can impact people in different ways, and dominant gendered norms are not seen as ideal by all. When ideals represent something that a person does not, or cannot, affiliate with, the experience is likely to be unhelpful. Thus, gender-based leisure can carry the risk that activities reflect limited notions of what it means to be a man (or woman).

In contrast, relatively little attention has been paid to female-centric activities. This is even though women are more likely to develop dementia, more likely to be carers and more likely to experience severe symptoms (Erol et al. 2015). Where limited research has considered gendered identities of women living with dementia, it has focused on aspects of appearance. For example, possession of a handbag, make-up and haircare are all associated with women living with dementia upholding a gendered sense of identity (see Sandberg 2018). Yet such a focus could reinforce a notion that femininity is centred on appearance and aesthetics. Furthermore, the gender imbalance apparent in many community groups, where most attendees and staff are female, fuels both the rationale behind designing male-centric services (as above), and underpins an assumption that groups are therefore appropriate for women (Savitch et al. 2015). Yet women are not a homogenous group, and a potentially harmful consequence of such an assumption is that a woman failing to engage in a social group environment might be seen as an individual problem, whereas the failure of a man to engage in a similar environment might be framed as a problem with the opportunity. This demonstrates how gender-based assumptions can impact how we interpret different people's engagement in leisure. Furthermore, it demonstrates how people living with dementia (and older people in general) might find their sense of individual identity diminished by overly simplistic binary stereotypes. Participation in leisure can be a key opportunity for the challenging and renegotiation of stereotypes, thereby promoting opportunities that better represent the diversity of men and women living with dementia. However, this is only likely if we critically explore the assumptions that shape the leisure opportunities on offer.

Sport reminiscence: an example of gendered leisure

I now turn to my ethnographic study of women's experiences of sport reminiscence activity for people living with dementia (Oatley 2021). Sport reminiscence involves using sport-related experiences to trigger memories and conversation. This is thought to be an enjoyable and sociable activity that helps people to share aspects of their identity, demonstrate skill and develop a sense of group belonging. As sport reminiscence often makes use of memories from the past, it is thought to be a suitable activity for people with the short-term memory loss that is common in dementia. In this way, sport reminiscence is a strengths-based leisure activity capable of reinforcing a positive sense of self and agency. In turn, this can provide an effective opportunity for citizenship. As a leisure activity, reminiscence is particularly useful to consider, as memories can also demonstrate ways in which gender shapes opportunities across the life-course, as well as how an individual's sense of gendered identity might change across time.

However, the rationale underpinning sport reminiscence is rooted in the assumption of a natural connection between men and sport described above. Indeed, it has largely been studied in men. It might be more appropriate to suggest that sport reminiscence has been promoted as an enjoyable and sociable activity that helps *men* to share aspects of their identity, demonstrate skill and develop a sense of group belonging.

Using ethnographic methods, I collected qualitative data from women affected by dementia using in-depth individual interviews, field conversations and observations at four sport reminiscence groups hosted by professional sports teams. All individual and group identities have been anonymized using pseudonyms.

Examples from this research illustrate how gender can impact on leisure opportunities for people affected by dementia. They demonstrate how the actions and behaviours of people can construct and uphold traditional gendered norms, even when the women's own experiences were contradictory. This demonstrates how rigid traditional gendered norms can be. However, examples also demonstrate how gendered norms can affect people in different ways and leisure can provide a context in which one's sense of identity is supported, reinforced or transformed.

Gender stereotypes

Findings from my research demonstrated that the sport reminiscence group was one in which a male-centric gendered context was constructed and reinforced. The four groups in the research represented professional football (soccer) and rugby clubs. This reflects the male dominance of professional sport in the UK. Reminiscence in each group was largely focused on the club's sporting history, despite many participants (male and female) identifying little connection to the club. Women reported that the primary reason for attending the sport reminiscence groups (usually, but not always, with their male partner) was the opportunity that groups promised for social interaction, demonstrating that leisure opportunities can be a key response to the risk of loneliness apparent in older age. There was never any focus on women's sport-related history, and this aligned with the common assumption that sport has historically been an activity centred on men.

It was common for women themselves to express attitudes that reinforced traditional gender-based stereotypes. The following examples demonstrate this, the first based on observations recorded at a group within a football club:

The women were gathered around a table talking about Christmas shopping. One of the women said, 'The women sit and gossip, while the men sit and talk about football!' Individual responses corroborated this. For example Marie, a woman living with dementia, recounted her feelings about how others attending a reminiscence group perceived the sport in question: 'Not a lot of women are interested in rugby ... they don't understand it.' Meanwhile Sandra, a care partner, said, while participating at a reminiscence group: 'I don't like women's boxing. That's too dangerous.'

Such views suggested that men are stimulated and knowledgeable about sport, while women are keener on domesticity and should avoid violence. These views reinforced traditional binary roles for men and women, strengthening sport as a masculine domain. A further example during an interview with Sarah, a daughter care partner, demonstrated how gender could intersect with other social characteristics (in this case, age) to reinforce cultural beliefs: 'Most women of the generation now experiencing dementia know sport arenas and the sporting atmosphere in a very different way to how a man knows it. ... I would say probably 90 per cent of men's heart rates will race, being in that environment, hearing that crowd.'

Stereotypical views expressed by women reinforced the notion that the typical sports fan was male, and thus, by virtue of being the 'other', women were assumed unlikely to have experiences of interest.

In the research I found it was rare for any women to participate in group sport reminiscence discussions, but in one-to-one interactions women often did reveal relevant childhood experiences. For example, Kath, a care partner told me: 'My Dad always went to watch Rovers. So, when I was seven, I was the one that went with him. I went to all the football games with Dad.' Anne, a woman living with dementia, recounted how she used to go to [football stadium] with her brother when she was a girl. She continued, 'It used to be 5 pence to get in, but 4 pence if you went to the pictures, so we used to do that!'

Thus, women's reluctance to contribute during sport reminiscence activities did not seem explained by a lack of relevant life experiences, but rather due to a context in which the women did not feel their experiences were relevant. Early life experiences were in contradiction to ideas that sport, and particularly football, has been a domain exclusively attended by men (and boys).

One way in which women did identify an interest in sport was through comments that recognized sportsmen as objects of sexual desire. Here, for example, is part of an interview I conducted with Pamela, a former care partner, who attended a reminiscence group at her local football club: 'But what changed my mind was rugby players. [We] went on a cruise to Samoa. The man who was our tour-guide ... Mike. He was a rugby player and I thought, "Yes!" [winks and laughs]'. A further example is provided by Sandra (a care partner) who attended another group based within a different club: 'I don't really understand rugby, but I think it's just the men. I like a bit of meat on the bone!'

By highlighting physical attraction to male athletes, the women reinforced narrow narratives of both gender and sexuality. The performance of a heteronormative narrative (where women admire the ideal man) upholds the privileged male stereotype, and a non-threatening female stereotype. Sport fandom based on physical attraction is generally dismissed as inauthentic, and thus does not threaten the masculine hegemony (the privileged male dominance). This heteronormative narrative can also work to *other* participants whose identities vary from such limited stereotypes of men, women and heterosexual sexuality. Just as disability-based assumptions might work to *other* people living with dementia (for example, an assumption that a person living with dementia will not understand instructions, and therefore the care partner is addressed and the person with dementia is *othered*), gender or sexuality-based norms could also create a leisure environment that becomes exclusive.

Actions of those facilitating the reminiscence could also reinforce the male-centric culture of activity:

> Daniel asked people to name a player from the era of the leather ball. Most people read out the player card in front of them. The exception was a male care partner and Sandra. Daniel noted that Sandra has knowledge. He didn't note the exception of the man having knowledge. (Field notes, Tunstead FC Group)

The fact that Daniel did not comment on the exceptional nature of the male care partner having knowledge suggested that he held preconceptions about who might, and who might not, hold knowledge. In this case, it was deemed noteworthy to recognize Sandra's knowledge, but not the male's similar behaviour.

In a second example, taken from my field notes gathered at a reminiscence group held within a football club, the deliberate targeting of men for participation in discussion suggests an underlying assumption about who holds the memories activities are intended to trigger: 'Leon asked who remembers [the family zone] and no one answered. He then asked each male participant directly. Most men simply nodded or shook their head. He did not ask any female participants.'

Both examples echo findings from a study of football reminiscence where care home staff assumed that the activity was for men, and thus, biased the sample of people offered the opportunity (Schofield and Tolson 2010). This demonstrates how gender-based assumptions can shape the way in which one is offered opportunities to participate, and the way in which social interaction occurs.

The risks of idealized characteristics

Another way in which gendered norms were reinforced in the sport reminiscence context was through the themes celebrated in the sport-related memories and activities. For example, people often used language focused on typical masculine ideals (e.g. toughness, strength) while simultaneously degrading qualities that might be more typically associated with feminine ideals, as this example given by Julie (the daughter of a man living with dementia and his care partner) illustrates: 'Here, it is tough men. They just keep going and going, they never want to come off that pitch.' Reflections I recorded offered additional examples:

> 'It was proper football in those days, proper football', said one man.
>
> Leon agreed: 'Yes, you actually were allowed to tackle then, players just wear slippers now.'
>
> 'And all these coloured boots', said the same man. 'They are more worried about the pretty colour of their boots than getting stuck in!' (Field notes, Dewhurst FC Group)

The language contributed to the construction of the 'ideal man' as tough and strong. In a leisure environment this can present barriers to participation if the person does not (or cannot) relate to such values. In the research, there was evidence from some female care partners who found that comparisons between former physical prowess and the current experience of dementia could be painful. For example, Helen, a care partner said: 'We did a game [of bowls] on Monday evening. It was pairs. I did it with someone else. He just sat and watched. He can't do it any more.' My field notes recorded another example from a care partner:

> Harriet spoke about her husband. Greg had been a great runner and she described his training efforts. But she also contrasted it with the sadness she feels now at his current condition.

These examples demonstrate that recalling former experiences can reinforce a sense of loss. This might be particularly true in a context such as sport, where idealized characteristics are often inextricably linked to youth. Idealized characteristics that might have been a part of past identity are not always attainable (for example, due to age, dementia or physical ability). For some people, focus on such ideal (but unattainable) characteristics might serve to undermine their identity by highlighting things they are no longer able to do. Although no examples were found in the study, it is just as possible that a person living with dementia might experience a similar discord if the leisure location in which they engage triggers a sense of failure, or loss of identity (be that gendered or otherwise). While the above examples relate more to age and disability than gender, they give a good example of the way in which particular values can serve to exclude or undermine people, rather than offer a positive opportunity to experience citizenship through the sense of being valued as a human being beyond being a person with dementia.

Women's meaningful connections to sport

Despite the apparent inflexibility of gendered identities in the sport reminiscence groups, many women identified their own meaningful connections to sport through one-to-one conversation with me. Some connections were to sport-related activities more commonly associated with women, as Pamela (a care partner) reflected: 'I was into netball. I used to love netball. I used to play for the school and county. That was my game.'

For other women, in addition to those above who had early experiences of attending sporting events, connections to sport could be through activities that were more usually considered male. For example, Carol (a woman living with dementia) said: 'It was rugby I wanted to play! And I did once. At school. We played mixed against the boys' grammar.' Meanwhile, I recorded the following extract in my research field notes after a conversation with Linda (a care partner): 'I really like watching snooker. My father-in-law used to say, "You can't like snooker, you're a woman". But I do. I don't play it, but I love to watch it. Have done for years.'

These examples demonstrate that while it is often assumed that women's connections to traditional male sports are a recent phenomenon, there is increasing evidence to the contrary (see Toffoletti 2017). Women's histories in sport have been hidden and the lack of visibility reinforces (and is reinforced by) gender-based assumptions within the sporting environment. In turn, this means that (particularly) older women might not always be offered opportunities to take part in sport as leisure because of the belief that they will have no interest or relevant life experience.

The research did find a common pattern of sport-related opportunity for many women. For example, several recalled that school-age participation reflected peak opportunity to participate in physical activity as leisure, and this often ceased upon marriage and childbirth. Thus Pamela, a former care partner, related: 'We got married and then we moved to Dewhurst. I didn't know any [netball] teams there. Then we had the boys.' I noted the following in my field notes: Mary (a care partner) told me she was captain of the school hockey team. But on leaving school, there weren't many opportunities to play. She then met Don, got married and had kids. 'He played a lot of football. And guess who washed the kit?!'

After marriage, many women noted that their relationship with sport would often continue through work done to enable other family members to participate (as player or spectator). Examples of support behaviour included providing childcare, transport, refreshments and doing the laundry. Such activities reflect traditional domestic labour division in the UK – for example, that a man might go to work to provide for his family, while a woman is responsible for childcare and domestic chores. This distinction constructs women's engagement in sport (and, more broadly, leisure time) as framed through servicing the needs of others. It also demonstrates how gendered expectations can change with age. In effect, men (and children) can seek out leisure activities, while a woman might find little opportunity as her time is consumed by fulfilling childcare and domestic responsibilities. Such a social construction can impact on an older woman's willingness to prioritize her own leisure time, as well as the value that others place on providing her with the opportunity for leisure. These norms reinforce a feminine duty to care for others. For some women, this might be a valued and important part of their identity. However, a narrative reinforcing a feminine duty of care might be unhelpful for those women who are struggling with such tasks. Indeed, the feminine pressure 'to care' might feel oppressive. This traditional stereotyping might be more likely in a leisure environment (such as football) that conforms to limited binary gender distinctions. In practice, this could create pressure for women to support their partner's access to leisure regardless of the impact that it might have on themselves. Indeed, there were women in the research who attended sport reminiscence groups for the benefit of their partner, but who were honest about their dislike of the sporting environment or (as above) found recalling their husband's former sporting prowess reinforced a sense of loss.

The varied ways in which gender-based assumptions affect individuals

The following examples, both taken from my research, demonstrate how gender-based assumptions affected individual women differently.

Example 1: Ruth

Ruth was in her eighties and living with dementia. Her sporting life has been relatively unaffected by gender-based norms. She began riding motorbikes with her brothers as a teen, was a champion motor racer, and won international awards for her exploits.

Ruth continues to be heavily connected with racing. It is an important part of her identity and leisure time. Her biography is inextricably bound up with that of her husband (Richard) and wider family. Richard's wholehearted acceptance and support of Ruth as a remarkable and successful female racer, (as well as wife and mother), meant that there was little discord between different aspects of her identity that might more usually have been associated with opposing gendered stereotypes. That is not to say that she was unaware of gender, but rather, her relationship with sport seemed unaffected by classic norms.

Researcher: How do you think the men that you were racing against felt losing to a woman?
Ruth: They were all right actually. They were quite good weren't they? There were never no animosity with them. They were all friends, you know. Whether it's because I was a woman and they, you know, I don't know.
Richard: She became one of the mukkas.
(Ruth (living with dementia) and Richard (husband), interview, Ashbourne FC Group)

In contrast to Ruth, Carol was one of several women in the research who showed awareness of gendered sporting stereotypes.

Example 2: Carol

Carol is in her early sixties and lives with an atypical dementia that primarily affects her language and communication. At first, she was reluctant to identify herself as 'sporty' and felt unsure if her experiences were relevant to the study saying: 'Not a lot! Not very sporty' [points at self].

Across three interviews, Carol described many connections with sport. This included watching her brother play rugby and cricket, playing hockey into her thirties, running, providing medical support to men's football teams, long-distance walking and being a keen spectator of international sport events (e.g. the Olympics, Wimbledon and cricket). In particular, she recalled wanting to play rugby (like her brother), and reflected on her enjoyment of hockey:

Carol: Maybe… I think… hockey's a bit like rugby… in…
Researcher: In physicality?
Carol: Physicality! Yes!
Researcher: And aggression?
Carol: Mmm… although not… yes… there's aggression, and there's aggression! (Carol, living with dementia, interview)

Carol would often laugh when describing her own personality characteristics that were more typical of sporting hegemonic masculinity. For example, her competitiveness, toughness and willingness to get hurt:

Researcher: Are you also competitive or...?
Carol: [Crosses her hands in her lap, looks down, embarrassed laugh, draws in breath, and looks back up] Mmm... [Shakes her head and laughs]... I could say no... but... I think I have realized [laughs and nods]
Researcher: Shall I reframe this? Would your friends say you're competitive?
Carol: [Mouths yes and nods vigorously]. Oh dear... [looks down and laughs]
(Carol, living with dementia, interview)

Carol reflected that she enjoyed hockey because it was 'tough and you haven't got to mind getting hurt!' Carol also laughed when suggesting that she didn't particularly enjoy netball at school because she felt there were too many rules, and it was, 'a bit soft'. Carol's suggestion was that such restraint was exactly why she did not enjoy it, but the admission was framed by embarrassed laughter, revealing an awareness that she had contravened traditional gendered norms.

Carol is an example of many of the women in the research who were familiar with sporting gender-based norms, and yet her own experiences were inconsistent with such norms. In the context of leisure and dementia, overlooking such diversity could result in activities that are only offered to, or taken up by, certain people.

Sport reminiscence: the opportunity to renegotiate gender stereotypes

Through her participation in the research, Carol began to reflect and reframe her competitive nature in terms she was more comfortable with.

The sport, hockey, walking the marathon. About who I am. [Mimes walking] Good. Better than others ... but for me, [organizing], writing, [I need] support. Practical, the art – I couldn't do it on my own now. All those, church, planning carol [service]. All these things not so good. But, walking is great, is better. I can do it. I can still achieve.

(Carol, a woman living with dementia, interview)

Thus, one-to-one sport reminiscence became a context through which Carol could recognize and share aspects of her identity that helped her to continue to live as well as possible. Although social norms that relate toughness to masculinity had made her reticent to begin with, her continued engagement in sport reminiscence through the research reconstructed the sport-related context into one that was better aligned with her sense of identity. It was also enjoyable and transformative in both helping her to understand her own strengths and needs and to share these with those around her. In effect, it enabled Carol to recognize that some of the more typically masculine characteristics she saw in herself were part of who she is, and part of how she can live well with dementia. Her toughness and competitiveness drive her to continue to achieve in sport-related activity and thus, for Carol (and others like her), leisure opportunities that enable her to continue to participate are crucial to her citizenship, her sense of identity beyond that of a person with dementia and continued pursuit of life goals.

Carol's story demonstrates that sport can be a powerful context through which to explore identity, but only when the context in which the exploration happens (in this case, one-to-one conversation) allows negotiation away from rigid social stereotypes. The reminiscence opportunity enabled Carol to reflect upon her own ongoing sense of identity (of which gender was a part), and how she continued to live well. In addition, it is a valuable example of how *doing* leisure (in Carol's case, walking) can be valuable experience that capitalizes on the strengths she has, again reinforcing her social citizenship. Carol's example is notable both in demonstrating how leisure can be life-enhancing, but also in how gendered identities are open to negotiation. This is important to consider, because however strong dominant norms are, they are not fixed, but open to negotiation if the right circumstances and context are available.

So what does this mean in practice?

For those supporting or enabling the involvement in leisure of people living with dementia

- Gender influences all aspects of life, and leisure is no exception. Leisure provides a location where people can experience a sense of gendered identity. Gender can affect who is offered opportunities, who takes up opportunities and how a person's engagement is interpreted and valued.

- Gender-based stereotypes within a particular culture can be rigid and continuously reinforced through language and behaviours of individuals and groups – for example, the idea that men are tough, strong and enjoy football. However, gendered identities are not binary, and are open to development. Dominant norms are not fixed, but open to renegotiation if the right circumstances are available.

- Participation in leisure can allow for negotiation away from limited stereotyping and provide opportunities for people to experience gender in ways that feel aligned to their sense of self. Rather than large-scale approaches to leisure based on broad stereotypes, offering people choice and control over leisure activities is fundamental to person-centred practice and the social citizenship of people affected by dementia.

For people living with dementia or their informal or family carers

- Gender – what it means to feel like a man, a woman or non-binary – can be an important part of identity and can influence which leisure activities a person chooses to take part in, and who they choose to take part in activities with.
- In this way, leisure can provide opportunities to experience and maintain a sense of gendered identity. In turn, this can help to support an ongoing sense of self.

For researchers

- The impact of gender and related power dynamics has been largely overlooked in dementia research. Often research designs, findings and activities for people affected by dementia have reinforced binary notions of what it means to be an older man or a woman.
- Gender can also influence how people's actions and interactions are interpreted and evaluated. More research into the impact of gender is vital to developing understanding of how gender can affect the lived experience.

References

Anstiss, D., Hodgetts, D. and Stolte, O. (2018) Men's re-placement: Social practices in a Men's Shed, *Health and Place*, 51: 217–23.

Carone, L., Tischler, V. and Dening, T. (2014) Football and dementia: A qualitative investigation of a community-based sports group for men with early onset dementia, *Dementia*, 15(6): 1358–76.

Clark, M., Murphy, C., Jameson-Allen, T. and Wilkins, C. (2015) Sporting memories and the social inclusion of older people experiencing mental health problems, *Mental Health and Social Inclusion*, 19(4): 202–11.

Erol, R., Brooker, D. and Peel, E. (2015) *Women and Dementia: A Global Research Review*. London: Alzheimer's Disease International.

Gleibs, I.H., Haslam, C., Jones, J.M. et al. (2011) No country for old men? The role of a 'gentlemen's club' in promoting social engagement and psychological wellbeing in residential care, *Ageing and Mental Health*, 15(4): 456–66.

Oatley, R. (2021) From washing boots to motor racing champions: Women's experiences of sport reminiscence activities for people affected by dementia. PhD thesis, University of Worcester.

Sandberg, L.J. (2018) Dementia and the gender trouble? Theorising dementia, gendered subjectivity and embodiment, *Journal of Aging Studies*, 45(6): 25–31.

Sass, C., Surr, C. and Lozano-Sufrategui, L. (2021) Expressions of masculine identity through sports-based reminiscence: An ethnographic study with community-dwelling men with dementia, *Dementia*, 20(6): 2170–87.

Savitch, N., Abbott, E. and Parker, G. (2015) *Dementia: Through the Eyes of Women*. York: Joseph Rowntree Foundation.

Schofield, I. and Tolson, D. (2010) *Scottish Football Museum Reminiscence Pilot Project for People with Dementia: A Realistic Evaluation*. Glasgow: Glasgow Caledonian University.

Toffoletti, K. (2017) *Women Sport Fans: Identification, Participation, Representation*. New York: Routledge.

5 Communication in social leisure activity

Joseph Webb

Summary

Much of the support offered to people who are newly diagnosed with dementia is in group settings, like memory cafes, day centres and activity groups. These groups are often focused on providing and supporting leisure activities like gardening, singing, art and doing quizzes. They are run by staff who aim to support people living with dementia to participate in various activities in ways that are accessible and adapted to them. Taking part in leisure activities in these settings is made possible by staff and people living with dementia talking to each other and doing activities together. Conversations between them can 'make or break' taking part in an activity. This chapter looks closely at communication, and specifically at how people living with dementia are supported to take part in leisure activities. It shows that activities of this kind can be opportunities for people living with dementia to participate as equals. It also shows that the success of an activity rests jointly on the staff member and the person living with dementia. Individual leisure activities themselves are not 'good' or 'bad' for people living with dementia. Instead, much depends on how people are supported and how the activity is tailored to the competencies of those taking part. Activities work best when they are done *with*, not *on*, people living with dementia.

Communication in social care leisure activities

Engaging in activities can be a vital part of 'living well with dementia' (Roberts 2011). However, some symptoms of dementia can mean that people living with dementia require support from others to be involved, to retain involvement (Phinney 2006) or to compensate for memory issues (Williams et al. 2019). Thus, 'leisure activities' can become essentially relational. Additionally, social care settings (activity groups, day centres, memory cafes, etc.) can become a key point at which leisure activities are accessed by people living with dementia. These activities are often in the form of 'staff-led' structured programmes such as quizzes, exercise or handicrafts (Webb et al. 2020). Whether the person benefits from taking part in leisure activities depends on their needs being realized and supported socially, often by staff members. It therefore makes sense to study such activities as social, and to look at the way that communication works within them. This chapter considers how aspects of communication might support or impede the full participation of people living with dementia in leisure of this kind.

It is important to look at what *really* happens when staff and people living with dementia interact. That is why this chapter draws on ten hours of video data of naturally occurring interactions between 28 people living with dementia and their conversation partners (often staff members) in five settings (two memory cafes, an activity group and two day centres). It was common in all settings for organized activities, such as quizzes, dancing, singing and gardening groups, to take place. I collected the data as part of a larger study about disabling and enabling social practices (Williams et al. 2023) for people with various disabilities in different settings. In this project I worked with co-researchers living with dementia who watched and commented on the videos. I refer at times in this chapter to their expertise about how the people in the videos may be feeling. The study followed a strict protocol approved by the Social Care Research Ethics Committee in the UK to ensure that people assessed as lacking capacity to consent had personal consultees who could advise on their behalf. All names are anonymized.

In reporting on what I found, I draw on a mixture of insights derived through visual ethnography (Pink 2001) as well as closer focus on the details of interaction derived from the principles of conversation analysis (Sidnell and Stivers 2012). Conversation analysis begins with the recording of naturally occurring interactions which are then transcribed in detail. A key insight from conversation analysis is that talk is organized into sequences (such as question – answer, offer – acceptance/refusal). Where one person starts a sequence (for example, by asking a question), they then shape and constrain what is possible for the next speaker. Here, we will look at these sequences, and at what actions speakers are accomplishing through their words.

I present below a series of vignettes that show real observed moments. For each there is an extract of conversational text between people taking part, and a description of the context and actions that occurred around this text. After each section, I sum up what impeded or supported communication. At the end of the chapter, these are summarized into learning points.

A quick note: this chapter will refer to 'first position' where a person goes first in a conversation (e.g. when they ask a question), and second position to refer to the turn that is shaped by the prior turn (e.g. when a person answers a question). Although conversation analysis is technical in nature, this chapter is intended to be accessible to a wide audience. Therefore, transcripts are presented in a straightforward way, and care has been taken to use non-technical language. The numbers in brackets represent the pauses and silences in seconds that occur during the interaction, and full stops in brackets like this (.) denote a brief silence of less than 0.1 of a second.

Including and excluding people with dementia from activities

A generic activity involving people living with dementia, such as a quiz, can be done in different ways. These permutations might make the difference between someone being included, or unintentionally being excluded from it. The following examples, featuring the same player, Pat, will show how someone living with dementia might have two very different experiences of taking part in a quiz.

Pat, who is in her early eighties and has dementia, is doing a quiz with her daughter Mel and her 'dementia navigator' (or support worker), Ann. We join the group as they engage in a quiz about famous crimes and criminals throughout history. The extract begins with the group discussing a possible answer to a question about the location of a famous historic prison. Lyn, a service centre organizer, walks behind them and leans over the table between Mel and Ann. The four players are in a line, with Pat on the far right. All the players look at a quiz sheet on the table in front of Mel.

An example of Pat being excluded from a quiz

Extract 5.1

1	Mel:	So. (1) Let's have a think about this other prison then.
2		(1.5)
3	Mel:	Is there one in France?
4		(15.4)
5		*(Lyn walks over and stands between Pat and Ann)*
6	Lyn:	It's a really hard quiz.
7		(2.8)
8		*(Mel turns over the quiz paper. Lyn bends over to*
9		*look at the quiz paper too.)*
10	Lyn:	I think you're probably right with number eight.

Extract 5.1 is a snippet of a long conversation in which the group try to answer difficult quiz questions, without engaging Pat in the activity. In the interaction, Pat sits forward trying to look at the quiz paper which sits in front of Mel. Eventually Pat slumps back in her chair and turns her head away from the others. No questions are addressed to Pat, and the position of the other three players without dementia mean that she is physically excluded from participating in the interaction.

Pat's slumping appears to be borne out of a response to her fellow-quizzers' numerous prior turns that exclude her from taking part. So how did Pat become excluded? First, the quiz questions were very specific (i.e. there was one answer to all questions – you either knew it or you did not). Secondly, the quiz questions were difficult and the group of players without dementia gave up asking Pat after the first two because Pat did not know the answers. Thirdly, the group wanted to complete the activity (i.e. answer all the questions), but this ended up excluding Pat from the task. Lastly, there were physical embodied ways of excluding Pat, such as the quiz sheet being far away from her, or through the other players turning away from Pat to look at each other. Thus, moving on with the activity licensed the exclusion of the sole player with dementia, as completing the activity took precedence over her inclusion.

How could Pat be included in the quiz?

From the example above, readers may wonder if Pat had any verbal language. Later in the day, the group had another quiz based around crime. However, this time there could be multiple answers to one question and players could draw on their life knowledge and experience to answer the questions, rather than trivia and fact recall alone. Mel and Pat have been given a quiz about personal safety, and what people can do to protect themselves from crime, in the home or out and about.

Extract 5.2

1	Mel:	What precautions can I take when meeting
2		friends in a coffee shop or a bar?
3		(2.1)
4	Pat:	Don't know the answer to that one.
5	Mel:	So what would you do with your personal
6		things? You don't really carry a handbag mum
7		do you.
8	Pat:	No.
9	Mel:	But what would you suggest I do
10		with my handbag?
11		(2.6)
12	Pat:	Take – take it out of view.

On lines 1–2, Mel poses a question read from the quiz sheet relating to safety precautions one could or should take when out at a coffee shop or bar. After a lengthy gap, Pat says 'Don't know the answer to that one.' Pat frames her non-answer as contingent; it is only this specific question which she cannot answer. On line 4 it would be perfectly conceivable for Mel to move to a subsequent quiz question. However, on lines 5–6, Mel reformulates the question to help Pat answer the question through providing additional information. This is further refined on lines 9–10 ('But what would you suggest I do with my handbag?'). Thus, Mel increases the specificity of the content and context of the question; in particular, she draws on their identities of 'mother' and 'daughter', where the former may be expected to give safety advice to the latter. Reformulating, or 'redoing', a question after a non-answer response is a way of making the question more understandable or easier to answer. After a silence, Pat gives a grammatically and topically fitted answer for how to keep the handbag safe.

So, what worked differently here? First, Pat could have given any number of answers to that question. There were many ways that Pat could answer, and therefore more chance she could participate. Secondly, because the question was not seeking one specific answer, Mel could reformulate the question to be about something Pat may have been more likely to answer; giving her daughter safety advice on where to keep her bag. Knowing Pat well made it easier for Mel to shift the question to being within Pat's experience. This is not to suggest that quizzes should avoid questions with a single answer, but that staff should consider tailoring the quiz to the competencies of the players. Lastly, in the first extract the players without dementia became focused on answering the quiz question, but that ended up leaving Pat out.

How to support reminiscence talk

It was common to see staff members talking with a person living with dementia about their memories. This could be as part of a formalized activity, where staff used meaningful objects (photos of the past, objects that may have some resonance in the person's life, etc.) to instigate and spark a conversation, or emerge more informally. Talking about one's life is deeply linked with identity and can be a meaningful and enriching experience wherein interactions with others may help to maintain the teller's worth and 'personhood'. However, not all strategies staff used to engage people in talking about the past were equally successful in leading to ongoing conversations.

For example, 'opener' questions often lead to trouble. A frequent form of opener was a 'Do you remember?' or 'Can you remember?' question, designed to orient the recipient to some aspect of their own experience.

Strategies for talking about the past which close down the conversation

Extract 5.3

1	Meg:	I wanted you to tell me a bit about what
2		you used to do for your job.
3		(0.8)
4	Sandra:	Can you remember,
5		(1)
6	Sandra:	when you were employed, what
7		your job was?
8	Jim:	Work *(laughs)*

Sandra prefaces her 'Can you remember?' with an explicit instruction to direct Jim to what he should talk about – namely, his job. Although 'Can you remember?' has the shape of a yes/no question, the phrase acts an indirect question to account for the possibility that Jim will in fact not be able to remember. It should be noted, however, that the formulation 'Can you remember, when you were employed, what your job was?' alludes to potential memory failure, as contrasted with 'I wanted you to tell me a bit about what you used to do for your job.' The former positions Jim as a potentially unreliable storyteller.

In the event, Jim delivers the non-conforming response 'Work' with a slight laugh. It may be that Jim does not remember and is using the generalized term 'Work' as a face-saving strategy. When the matter to be remembered specifically relates to the life of the recipient, and their ability to remember is called into question, this can lead to a complex and sensitive negotiation of 'Who knows what?', as the person living with dementia is put in the position of perhaps not being able to recall details of their life that they are being questioned about, and that one might normally be expected to know.

Another potential issue is that staff know a lot about the person living with dementia and their life, possibly through previous conversations, that the person may not recall in the present conversation. However, if the staff member leads the conversation with a series of questions designed to elicit information they already know the answer to, the person living with dementia is 'put on the spot'. This can look more like a test than a shared conversation. Here, we see John, a man living with dementia, talking to Bob, a staff member at a day centre.

Extract 5.4

1	Bob:	Who are you married to John? What's
2		your wife's name?
3	John:	Sandra.
4	Bob:	Sandra, that's right.

The conversation begins with Bob, the staff member, asking John who he was married to. Before John can answer, Bob asks a follow-up question: 'What's your wife's name?' Even at this early juncture we can see that there are assumptions in these questions that suggest Bob knows the answer already; for example, he is assuming that John is married. If Bob really did not know, it would be more socially normative to ask the person *if* they were married. Bob's prior knowledge of John's wife is revealed after John gives his wife's name on line 3, and Bob confirms the validity of the answer ('Sandra, that's right'). This evaluative third turn (after the question and answer) is commonly seen in teacher–student interactions, where teachers ask students 'known answer questions'. This matters because it can resemble a test, rather than a conversation between equals.

While asking questions of John is one way of getting a response and possibly getting a conversation going, it leaves him with little he can do other than provide the right answer, or say he does not know. This is unlikely therefore to lead to a shared and equal conversation, as the staff member is always 'in the driving seat'. Additionally, asking questions which are retrospectively revealed to be 'known answer questions' can make the conversation look more like a test, where answers are appraised. Attempts to encourage reminiscence through questions where one person is seeking the 'right' answer may not lead to a conversation in which each person has equal power.

How to use knowledge of the person to talk about the past successfully

In the following extract, we will see Rob, a man living with dementia, talking to Jan, a staff member, about his piano playing. Knowing that Rob was a keen musician, Jan had brought over some sheet music to show Rob. This meaningful object was used by Rob as way to talk about playing the piano, and it elicits some memories. Lots of the conversation is led by Rob, rather than Jan asking questions for Rob to confirm. Unlike the attempt to launch in with a 'Do you remember?' question, Rob's identity as a piano player has been roundly emphasized throughout the interaction. Jan has spent some time showing Rob some piano music, and asking him what the notes mean, when she finally asks him a specific question about his memories on lines 26–31.

Extract 5.5: Doing inclusive reminiscence talk

1	Rob:	It's called playing the ivories.
2	Jan:	*(moves her hands as if playing the piano)*
3	Jan:	Play – tinkling the ivories yeah.
4	Rob:	And we know where the ivories come from.
5	Jan:	Yeah er African – African elephants.
6	Rob:	Yeah.
7	Jan:	Yeah (.) I don't think they do
8		I don't think they are made
9		of ivory any more. I think they're probably
10		just the old ones made of ivory row.
11	Rob:	*(nods head)* Yes, when we were in Kenya
12	Jan:	Yeah
13	Rob:	there was a concert or- organized by (.)
14		Er um (0.2) you know they all (.)
15	Jan:	Travel arrangements travel agents
16	Rob:	suddenly got (0.1) even the Queen when
17		she was there
18	Jan:	Yes
19	Rob:	and the – the girl guides
20	Jan:	Oh right

```
21   Rob:   em er and I was in the –
22   Jan:   Boy scouts yeah
23   Rob:   Yes (.) and er (0.1) you know they say
24          'give us a tune'
25          (plays with fingers as if on piano)
26   Jan:   Oooh Rob, you know when you
27          went to Kenya?
28   Rob:   Yes
29   Jan:   And you're saying about the Queen
30          in Kenya (.) Are you thinking of
31          Treetops?
32   Rob:   (.) Yes that's where they stayed at.
33   Jan:   Yeah, the Kenyan resort where the Queen stayed.
34          Did you go to Treetops?
35   Rob:   Well I (0.2) er the thing is that all my (0.3)
36          sepia (0.1)
37   Jan:   Yes
38   Rob:   photos are pretty awkward for me.
39   Jan:   Yes, to look at.
40   Rob:   And I played the piano (0.1) er and I I er
41          talked to er (.) the Queen.
42   Jan:   Yes (sits back with a smile)
43   Rob:   when she was a girl
44   Jan:   Yes
```

Rob's talk about 'playing the ivories' is taken up by Jan. Note that this is based on Rob's claim to greater knowledge not only about his own life but also about the terms and issues associated with the domain of piano playing. Then Rob says, 'And we know where the ivories come from.' The roles of questioner and respondent are then reversed as Jan provides a response to Rob's question, and her turn works around neatly to another turn slot for Rob, by her reference to 'just the old ones made of ivory now'. Rob's embodied yes (a nod) immediately takes this up, and he then shifts the topic to 'when we were in Kenya'. So far, what is remarkable in this extract is Rob's continued dominance of first-position turns. Down to line 26, Jan is constantly in second position and responding to Rob's talk, orienting to Rob's right to know about his own life and experiences. It is at line 26 that this changes where Jan says: 'Oooh Rob, you know when you went to Kenya? And you're saying about the Queen in Kenya (.) Are you thinking of Treetops?'

It is notable that Jan gives Rob a possible answer to the question within the question itself (that he is referring to Queen Elizabeth II staying at Treetops), while also giving Rob the right to confirm or disconfirm her point. It also comes after Rob has already raised the topic of Kenya and the Queen. Thus, the talk about Kenya, the Queen and Treetops emerge out of Rob's talk and follows his narrative cues. Rob is mostly in control of the conversation. When he is asked a question, Jan both refers to a previous conversation they may have had, and also gives Rob the answer to the question (Treetops) that requires a yes/no answer, rather than asking him a test-type question (i.e. Do you remember the name of the place the Queen stayed in Kenya?).

So, what worked differently here? Jan got the conversation going by introducing a meaningful object to Rob (piano sheet music) which allowed him to lead the conversation. Where Jan did ask a question, it was not done as a test, but referred to a past conversation which gave Rob the right to confirm or disconfirm her question, rather than asking him for specific information. In all the extracts, the staff show that they know the person well and have knowledge of their life. However, one should take care to make it a conversation, rather than turning it into a memory test.

Making space for interaction *within* activities

In this section I look at two different ways a quiz could be facilitated, and the implications this has for the involvement of people living with dementia. For example, in some quizzes players were chosen in order, by name, to answer a quiz question by a staff member (see Webb et al. 2020). While this guaranteed everyone got a chance to participate, it often resulted in players being put 'on the spot' and prevented other people living with dementia from taking part at the same time because it would intrude on the current player's turn.

One big quiz: staff controlling who can take a turn

Take the following example from a day centre for people living with dementia, in which players are asked to provide an answer that meets *two* conditions: a food beginning with the letter R. Here, each player is asked in turn to name something from a category that begins with a letter chosen by the quiz master. The extract features a staff member asking the questions and three players: Julie, Richard and Tim.

Extract 5.6

1	Staff:	Moving on, Richard. Can you think of a
2		food beginning with R?
3		(1.8)
4	Julie:	Radish huh huh ha huh huh.
5		(1.7)
6	Richard:	Potatoes
7		(2)
8	Staff:	Not quite have another go.
9	Tim:	Hmm, rump steak.

10	Staff:	Food beginning with R.
11		*(The staff members draws an R in the air with his fingers)*
12	Richard:	Oh, sorry huh huh huh huh huh.
13	Staff:	That's alright. Carry on?
14	Julie:	Oh me back.
15		(8)
16	?:	Oh wooo woo woo.
17		(2.1)
18	?:	(clears throat)
19		(2.2)
20	Tim:	Come on.
21	Richard:	Huh huh huh huh huh.
22	Tim:	Huh huh rice.
23	Julie:	Huh huh huh.
24		(0.6)
25	Richard:	No
26	Staff:	No? Okay then let's move on to Sal.

On line 1, Richard is selected by the staff member to answer a quiz question ('Can you think of a food beginning with R?'). Julie provides an answer 'out of turn' (line 4) which is not responded to by the staff member. Richard then gives an incorrect answer ('potatoes') to the question. Following a silence, the staff member confirms the inadequacy of the answer, and instructs Richard to 'have another go'. However, there are clear signs that Richard is unable to produce a relevant response (the delay in lines 3 and 5, and the incorrect answer in line 6). It could be seen as a kindness that Richard is given a second turn, but this also puts him in a vulnerable position where the prior sequence suggests he is struggling to answer the question.

Other players call out correct answers (lines 4, 9 and 22). Here, as in many other examples in the data, turns taken during someone else's go are ignored as if they were not spoken. This is perhaps not surprising as to acknowledge the correctness of the answer could be rude to Richard, as it is his turn. The out of turn correct answers in this extract could of course be understood as working to help Richard, who is not able to answer. Richard however does not treat them as such, and does not repeat or use one of the multiple correct answers as his own. Richard's long silence (lines 13–20) shows that answering the question remains difficult. Richard sits motionless for 15 seconds, in which time the silence is punctuated by an off-topic interjection from Julie (line 14).

Usually, when someone asks a question, we expect an answer to be forthcoming. When it is met by silence, this signals a problem. Often if a person does not know the answer to the question they provide a reason or rationale for being unable to do so. This may explain Tim's utterance ('come on') which is hearable as annoyance for Richard's silence which holds up the game. This elicits Richard's laughter in response (line 21). This whole time, it is Richard's turn to answer the quiz question. While his turn is held open by the staff member, the responsibility and pressure to provide a correct answer is also increased. He is 'put on the spot'; a situation he deals with by laughter.

A few things are notable about the quiz above: the first is that the people are divided into staff (who ask the questions), and people living with dementia, who are the players. This was seen by co-researchers living with dementia who collaborated on this project as potentially divisive. The second is that no one is allowed to speak other than the person whose turn it is. If they do, their turns are ignored. This prevents the game being particularly social. The third is that taking turns to be asked a question in front of a large group could be seen to put people on the spot. Lastly, there is no opportunity to do anything with the question other than to give a correct or incorrect answer, or cede one's go.

Small group quiz: players with dementia self-selecting to take a turn

An alternative way to organize a quiz was in small groups, with a staff member as part of the team. In this, a format where players were sitting around a table facing each other tended to work best. Let's look at an example.

We join the quiz players after an answer – 'telegram' – had been given to 'Name a form of communication beginning with the letter T'. The extract features Fred, Barbara and the staff member.

Extract 5.7

1	Staff:	What one do you like, team? What one shall we
2		go with?
3	Fred:	Thread.
4	Staff:	Yeah. Thread. I think telegram, because
5		they might not – the other team…
6	Fred:	Telegram, yeah.
7	Staff:	Yeah, telegrams. Let's go with that,
8		because that's an unusual one.
9	Barbara:	Yeah.
10	Fred:	Yeah, my father had a – used telegrams
11	Staff:	So do you remember getting telegrams? You
12		don't see that any more nowadays, do you,
13		people don't send telegrams.
14	Fred:	No, they – but…
15	Barbara:	Yeah, they would knock on the door with
16		a telegram, your heart started beating.
17	Staff:	Really?
18	Barbara:	And you, heh heh.
19	Staff:	Yeah, yeah you wondered.
20	Barbara:	What's wrong.

On lines 1–2 the staff member attempts to elicit a collective decision regarding which one of the previously given answers they should choose. Fred offers a new possible answer on line 3 ('thread'), and while the staff member acknowledges Fred's turn, she begins to give a reason for choosing 'telegram' as the answer. While the staff member treats herself as in charge, she is part of the group and tries to engage the players in a joint decision.

On line 10 Fred initiates a new action not related to answering the quiz question, informing the group that his father had used telegrams. This piece of information is treated as the beginning of a story, with the staff member probing Fred for additional information (line 11) while making an observation that builds upon this turn ('You don't see that any more nowadays, do you, people don't send telegrams.') Fred's initiation of the topic of telegrams then leads to Barbara sharing her own recollections about what it meant to receive a telegram when its content could be life altering (lines 15–16, 18), on which the staff member collaborates with her (line 19).

Here then we have two players building on topics in the quiz to share aspects of their lives. So, while quizzes are based on 'question and answer' sequences, in group quizzes played as a team there were more opportunities for players with dementia to use their turns to act in ways that did not expedite the completion of the quiz, but were of social value to them. This suggests that quizzes in these contexts may create opportunities for talk that appears divergent but can make the social occasion a bit richer, and allows opportunities for 'doing social capital', as the players position themselves as knowledgeable story tellers. This more informal approach meant there was space for these stories, and that the players were not 'taking someone else's turn', as in the previous extract.

So, what can we learn from this? Small group quizzes allowed players more agency in taking turns and actions that *they* initiated (e.g. telling the group about their experiences connected to telegrams) rather than being in second position, responding to quiz questions. Players could also say they did not know an answer and continue to be involved in the interaction. However, in mediated turn allocation quizzes, not knowing the answer meant losing one's right to take part (at least until their turn came around again). Lastly, staff members playing as part of the team can support conversations in a more informal way than when acting as a 'quiz master' with one-at-a-time question rounds. This shows the importance of engaging in activities as equals, a topic explored further in the following section.

Doing activities as equals

Activities where the staff participated with people living with dementia on an equal basis generally led to increased participation. Staff may need to direct the action to some degree, but it is still possible to do this while maintaining the jointness of the activity.

Take the following exchange from a gardening group in which Ron, a staff member, and Dan, a man living with dementia, are filling up a compost bin from the compost heap together. The extract starts with Ron and Dan walking over towards the compost heap.

Extract 5.8

1	Ron:	So like Lizzy said, we'll do a little bit
2	Dan:	Do some of it.
3	Ron:	just to get it going, and there's a lot of that
4	Dan:	Yeah.
5	Ron:	we can leave to rot down.
6	Dan:	Yeah.
7	Ron:	So do you want to take the lid off Dan?
8		(2)
9	Dan:	*(Walks over to the compost bin)* Top off, yep.
10	Ron:	Take the top off. Right, so if you get some of that
11		*(points to the top of the compost heap)* in
12	Dan:	Yeah. *(shovels the earth into the compost bin)*
13		*(skipping forward 30 seconds)*
14	Dan:	Can I have the fork? It's better with the fork.
15	Ron:	Yeah.
16	Dan:	Could be.
17	Ron:	Yeah. That's lovely, that woody material will be
18		nice for it.
19		*(Ron stands and watches Dan shovel the earth into*
20		*the compost bin)*
21		(10)
22	Ron:	I'll get a bit of grass. *(walks over to*
23		*the compost heap)*
24	Dan:	Yeah.
25	Ron:	I'll get a bit of grass.
26	Dan:	Bit of grass, yeah.
27	Ron:	Then you can (1.5) give it a good mix.
28		*(Dan shovels some grass)* That's it. Now if
29		you start stirring it up.
30	Dan:	Yeah right. Because the worms get in then.

The extract begins with Ron repeating what Lizzy, the person running the gardening group, said their task was: to fill the compost bin to 'get it going' and to leave the rest to 'rot down'. Notice how Ron frames this as a joint activity from the start by using 'we', while also reminding Dan of the task they will be doing. When Ron does give Dan instructions, he does so in a mitigated way that undercuts the presumption of giving an order – e.g. 'So do you want to take the lid off, Dan?' – which leaves agreement or disagreement up to Dan. Because the task is physical, there is a long stretch of silence while they are jointly engaged in the task (line 21). These types of silences were not treated as problematic when participants were engaged in a joint physical project, but they would be if they were sat looking at each other in a conversation (as in the reminiscence talk earlier on). Doing an activity together side by side can reduce the pressure to always be talking.

Ron is also careful to not only give instruction, but to engage in the task himself. For example, he walks off saying 'I'll get a bit of grass' to add into the compost bin that Dan is mixing up. This is affirmed by Dan: 'Bit of grass, yeah', showing his agreement. This hints at an equality between the two, Dan treating Ron's announcement of his next action as one that he has some say over. Dan is an active participant in the activity, helping to shape what happens next, and the activity is approached by both as something to be completed as equals. This jointness and equality of action is further shown by Dan responding to Ron's directive 'Now if you start stirring it up' with his own independent knowledge claim about why this is a good idea: 'Yeah right. Because the worms get in then' (Bartlett and O'Connor 2010).

Here we can see that, while Ron gives some instructions, he does so in such a way as to soften the social action by treating Dan as having the right to push back ('do you want to take the lid off?' rather than 'take the lid off', 'you can give it a good mix', rather than 'mix it'). Dan, for his part, also orients to the jointness of this shared activity by showing his own physical competency in the gardening task, as well as foregrounding his own knowledge (e.g. 'Can I have the fork? It's better with the fork' and 'Yeah right. Because the worms get in then').

Staff can run the risk of separating themselves from the people they support – for example, by enacting an activity for people living with dementia that they do not participate in, or by doing an activity *on*, rather than *with*, people living with dementia. Here, the task is framed as a collaborative activity, and the pair approach it as an activity to be jointly negotiated, with space for each of their expertise and turns at talk. Approaching the task as something to be enacted jointly supports the relational enactment of social citizenship, with Dan playing an active role in contributing to the task and being given opportunities to make choices about his participation in it (Bartlett and O'Connor 2010).

Doing activities together: suggestions for best communication practices

This chapter has examined how the enactment of leisure activities rests on the communication between people living with dementia and the staff who support them. I have shown that people living with dementia can play an active role in shaping their leisure activities, if given appropriate support to do so. Equally, activities may need to be adapted and reshaped by others to enable people with dementia to be active participants. Social citizenship is partly defined by camaraderie with others and participating in meaningful activities (Bartlett and

O'Connor 2010). We have seen that these are not abstract concepts but are talked into being in the to and fro of real interactions.

By looking at examples where similar (or the same) activities are done in different ways, this chapter has shown that it is not necessarily *what* the activity is that matters, but *the way* it is done, that can be important in supporting and engaging in activities with people living with dementia. For example, in some of the 'reminiscence talk', memory problems were foregrounded before they are interactionally relevant (e.g. 'Can you remember X?'). In this way the presumption of impairment or interactional inability can also impact the conversation. It is shown here that the difficulties in interaction are shared and jointly created – not something which solely resides within the domain of the person with a communication 'problem'.

Having a joint task, possibly aided by an object (gardening or talking about sheet music) can help facilitate a conversation and provide opportunities for camaraderie. However, ideally this should be led, or co-led by the person living with dementia. For example, objects can also be used as a resource to question a person living with dementia, and then the conversation becomes like a test. For example, we saw staff asking people living with dementia who people were in photographs, and then subsequently revealing they knew the answer to the question all along. Staff can avoid this by trying to not always occupy 'first position' (i.e. the one who asks questions), or to not show that the question they asked was in fact known all along (i.e. responding with 'that's right', or 'well done'). Where the object is related to an area of competence (as with Rob's sheet music in Extract 5.5, or Dan's gardening tools in Extract 5.8), it led to conversations around shared interests that are within the person living with dementia's expertise. Staff may need to adapt their approach in the moment to give instructions, hints or tips, but this can be done in a way that ensures success in the activity if the goal is jointly shared.

It is important for people without dementia to be responsive and adaptable so that they can reshape the activity in the moment in response to the needs of the person living with dementia. For example, questions could be reformulated if they were not understood the first time (as in Extract 5.2). Equally, space could be created within the activity itself so that people living with dementia could take turns at talk that was related to the topic at hand, but not necessarily the task (Extract 5.7). Where who could speak was more strictly prescribed (as in Extract 5.6), it meant that there was less chance for interaction from the wider group, and people's turns could be ignored because they came at the 'wrong time'. Where the aim is to encourage social interaction, this way of doing activities may work against that goal. In this research, I worked with co-researchers living with dementia who wanted to emphasize that people living with dementia could lead the activities themselves rather than the staff, and that this could make the activities feel less institutional. They saw the involvement of people with dementia as key to equalizing any potential power imbalances between staff and people living with dementia.

All examples showed that communication during leisure activities generally works best when staff and people living with dementia do the activity together, rather than the staff member doing the activity *on* or *for* the person living with dementia. This can help prevent institutional identities and deficit framings becoming entrenched. Despite the data being collected in social care settings, these observations have broader relevance for the inclusion of people living with dementia in leisure activities in any setting. Where power dynamics are tilted towards the person without dementia leading the activity, rather than doing it together, this can result in activities which close down opportunities for communication that is led by the person living with dementia.

By focusing on the details about communication, we can move away from the often presumed or assumed deficits of the person with dementia, towards the interactional strategies needed within a two-way conversation. This view helps to prevent us seeing difficulties in interaction as residing solely in the domain of the person with a communication 'problem', and towards empowering people with dementia by reframing any interactional difficulties as jointly created.

So what does this mean in practice?

For those supporting or enabling the involvement in leisure of people living with dementia

- Providing a group or shared activity is good because it can help people to take part at their own pace rather than feeling that they are being put on the spot.
- Be aware of making sure that you are doing activities *with* people. It is easy to take over, but that will defeat the object of engaging and connecting.
- Create as many opportunities as possible for participants with dementia to lead the conversation or activity. Capitalize on knowledge that you have about participants to ask them to talk about or show their knowledge about personally meaningful objects or topics.
- Use questions as a way of continuing the conversation, not 'testing' the person. This can be done by asking the person a question to confirm or disconfirm something.

For people living with dementia

- Joining others in group activity is a great way of building confidence. The person should choose how much to contribute.
- If the person living with dementia has knowledge or skills in an activity, then others will generally be very happy to hear their experiences. Speaking out or demonstrating something can give a real confidence boost.
- It's sometimes difficult to tell beforehand whether someone is going to enjoy a particular activity or not. If the person does not like the group, then no one should make them go again.

For family, friends and care partners

- Taking part in group activities is a good way to rebuild confidence and have some fun together. Decisions about how much each person wants to contribute should be made at the pace that suits those involved.
- If you know the person living with dementia has something to contribute then they may need gentle encouragement to help them to share.
- Be careful not to take over. It's easy to fall into answering for other people unless we take care not to.

References

Bartlett, R. and O'Connor, D. (2010) *Broadening the Dementia Debate: Towards Social Citizenship*. Bristol: Policy Press.

Phinney, A. (2006) Family strategies for supporting involvement in meaningful activity by persons with dementia, *Journal of Family Nursing*, 12(1): 80–101.

Pink, S. (2001) *Doing Visual Ethnography: Images, Media and Representation in Research*. London: Sage.

Roberts, K. (2011) Leisure: The importance of being inconsequential, *Leisure Studies*, 30(1): 5–20.

Sidnell, J. and Stivers, T. (2012) *The Handbook of Conversation Analysis*. Chichester: Wiley-Blackwell.

Webb, J., Lindholm, C. and Williams, V. (2020) Interactional strategies for progressing through quizzes in dementia settings, *Discourse Studies*, 22(4): 503–22.

Williams, V., Gall, M., Mason-Angelow, V. et al. (2023) Misfitting and social practice theory: Incorporating disability into the performance and (re)enactment of social practices, *Disability & Society*, 38(5): 776–97.

Williams, V., Webb, J., Dowling, S. and Gall, M. (2019) Direct and indirect ways of managing epistemic asymmetries when eliciting memories, *Discourse Studies*, 21(2): 199–215.

Realm Two

Time – how it is used and by whom

6 Understanding meaningful moments

Robyn Dowlen and John Keady

Summary

Music and the creative arts can help ground people living with dementia in the present moment. Research has shown that taking part in creative activity can enable a greater sense of choice, connectedness and belonging. However, there is little research that examines the role of everyday creativity as leisure in the lives of people living with dementia. A focus on 'in the moment' experiences can help to frame arts and cultural experiences as things that happen in the everyday. It can help to position creative arts as leisure activities. But it can be difficult for researchers to know how to understand and measure the value of fleeting creative moments and everyday creativity. We suggest that doing this requires an investment in the use and application of sensory and embodied methods, including the use of video technology. This chapter provides some examples of these and recommendations for researchers working in this area, arguing that such understanding will help support increased opportunities for people living with dementia.

Introduction

This chapter reports on research from the UK that has looked to explore what 'being in the moment' means in the context of creative arts experiences held by people living with dementia. The first author (Robyn Dowlen) completed her doctoral studies on the topic of 'in the moment' musical experiences within Manchester Camerata's *Music in Mind* programme (which will be outlined later in this chapter). The second author (John Keady) was the lead supervisor of this work and has a long history of using sensory and embodied methods to understand people living with dementia's 'in the moment' experiences. We have also co-authored several publications that have conceptualized 'moments' in the context of people living with dementia's everyday lives.

Interest in the role and meaning of creative arts as leisure activities for people living with dementia has grown significantly over the past 20 years. For instance, in the media there have been several powerful stories of the ways in which creative arts have supported people living with dementia to lead meaningful and fulfilling lives and connect to the here and now. Researchers have also begun to understand the significance of creative and cultural experiences for people living with dementia in studies exploring visits to museums and galleries, music programmes, devising theatrical performances centred on storytelling, painting, creative writing and dance, to name but a few. It is clear that many people living with dementia make time, or have time made for them, to undertake creative endeavours. However, less is known about the experiences of people living with dementia when they engage with the creative arts in their everyday lives.

This chapter provides an overview of research literature that explores the lived experience of people with dementia taking part in the arts, as well as examining the ways in which creativity contributes to how time is experienced by people living with dementia. With its roots in improvised music-making, we will also outline our conceptual framework for understanding 'in the moment' or 'here and now' experiences in the everyday lives of people living with dementia and link this to ideas and constructions of leisure activities (Keady et al. 2022).

Arts, creativity and dementia

To date, there is little research that examines the role of everyday creativity as leisure in the lives of people living with dementia (Bellass et al. 2019). The majority of research exploring the arts, creativity and dementia has been more concerned with the delivery and evaluation of creative arts activities as psychosocial interventions. It has been known for some time that people living with dementia have expressed a need to access everyday activities and patterns of life 'in ways that maximize [personal] choice and control' (Bamford and Bruce 2000: 553). This need for personal autonomy and agency has been highlighted by the activist Kate Swaffer (2015), a person living with dementia, who uses the term 'prescribed dis-engagement'™ to showcase the negativity that imbues professional 'advice' to prepare for a life of dependency and a loss of social role and function following a diagnosis of dementia. Arguably, this detrimental positioning risks diminishing the everyday citizenship of people living with dementia as the person's previous creative arts training, or experiences in creative arts programmes, may lead to their exclusion from arts-based research activities for fear that it might act as a 'confounding variable' in controlled trials. Consequently, existing research may not be giving a real picture of the range and depth of interests and experiences of arts and creativity of people living with dementia.

In contrast, the terms 'in the moment' and 'here and now' are becoming increasingly common in creative arts and dementia literature. Being 'in the moment' as it is related to people living with dementia has been defined in the following way:

> Being in the moment is a relational, embodied, and multisensory human experience. It is both situational and autobiographical and can exist in a fleeting moment or for longer periods of time. All moments are considered to have personal significance, meaning and worth. (Keady et al. 2022: 687)

A wealth of information can be gathered from examining creative experiences from an 'in the moment' perspective. For example, both family carers and healthcare professionals have reported that 'in the moment' musical experiences have value, noting that these do not lose their merit even if the perceived benefits for the person living with dementia do not last beyond the session time (Dowlen et al. 2018). A focus on 'in the moment' experiences that positions arts and cultural experiences as occurrences in the everyday invites us to explore creative arts as leisure activity with a role and value above and beyond any 'therapeutic' benefits. This reframing can help researchers and arts practitioners to better understand the creative arts as part of a person's leisure pursuits throughout their life, rather than purely an intervention at times of 'crisis' or as part of a planned activity, however important such events may be.

The following sections first provide a contemporary overview of 'leisure time' and its relationship to 'in the moment' experiences. We then present a conceptual model underpinning a moments-based approach to understanding arts and cultural leisure in the context of the lived experience of dementia. Next, we outline a case study drawn from an improvisation-based music programme for people living with dementia and their family carers. Finally, we contextualize what we have learned from this work by drawing on broader theories involving the creative arts as everyday leisure pursuits.

Time, moments and dementia

It is not possible to discuss being 'in the moment' or the 'here and now' without first examining lived experiences of time. The lives of many people living with dementia will be confined to the repetitive and regimented nature of 'clock time' where certain routines are performed at the same time, and in the same way, day after day. This experience can be faced by people with dementia living in supportive environments, such as in a care home, as well as at home. As a practical illustration, the authors of this chapter have been in live music sessions in care homes where staff removed percussion instruments from people's hands and replaced them with cups of tea because '11am signalled teatime'. This adherence to routine and clock time demonstrates how time pressures and heavy workloads placed on care staff (and family carers) can get in the way of providing meaningful 'in the moment' occupation for people living with dementia.

Moreover, care staff adherence to routines can also result in people living with dementia waiting around 'for something to happen', rather than being full and active partners in the care process with their everyday citizenship respected. This regimented following of clock time can lead to a sense of repetitiveness and dissatisfaction for people living with dementia. Indeed, it is rare to see the spaces created by following clock time framed as an opportunity for meaningful and productive engagement and interaction. This is regrettable because, as Dupuis and colleagues have shown earlier in this book, people living with dementia often find meaning in the 'ordinary' and 'everyday', with leisure activities providing opportunities for self-growth and personal enjoyment.

While there is not a significant amount of research exploring the subjective experiences of lived time for people living with dementia, there is a growing recognition of the idea of 'moments in time', and of how supporting a person living with dementia to live 'in the moment' could facilitate a greater sense of connectedness to oneself, to other people, and a greater grounding in both time and space (Keady et al. 2022). In everyday language, a moment can have a range of meanings and colloquial understandings, such as a 'moment to oneself', a 'lightbulb moment', a 'precious moment' or to live 'moment by moment'. What binds each of these understandings together is the recognition that a moment is transitory and exists in the present. Furthermore, as Mason (2018: 193) goes on to explain, moments may be charismatic not because they are measurable fractions of clock time, but because they are 'multisensory glimpses, windows, apertures, or revelations' into a person's everyday world and lived experience.

People living with dementia have also written about the significance of 'moments'. Christine Bryden, diagnosed with young-onset Alzheimer's disease at the age of 46, shared the following self-reflection in her first book, *Who Will I Be When I Die?* (1998: 144): 'I plan to enjoy each and every experience, even though I might not remember them from moment to moment – the experience of each moment will be enough for me.' This experience of being immersed 'in the moment' was further developed in her second book, in which she writes 'many of us seek earnestly for this sense of the present time, the sense of "now" of how to live each moment and treasure it as if it were the only experience to look at and wonder at' (Bryden 2005: 11).

If such descriptions of lived experience have merit, and it is difficult to discount given the authentic representations shared by people living with dementia, then 'in the moment' activity has personal significance, meaning and worth even though, for people living with dementia, such moments may not be fully remembered later because of memory difficulties. This lived experience builds on an idea of dementia as being a 'constantly fluid, dynamic and responsive series of moments which also has implications for the re-imagination of dementia care' (Smith et al. 2021: 7). By re-imagining the relationship between dementia, lived time and moments, it becomes possible to open up opportunities to dedicate some of these moments to meaningful and purposeful leisure, including through participation in the creative arts.

Moments of creativity

Reference to 'in the moment' or the 'here and now' are increasingly common in research about the arts, creativity and dementia. One reported benefit of participation in arts and creativity is that a full and enjoyable immersion in the activity does not rely on having a biographical memory. This means that during such interactive participation, people living with dementia are not necessarily judged, or limited, by the cognitive challenges that may affect them in other parts of their daily lives (Ward et al. 2021). Engagement with the arts, especially activity that is participatory in nature, affords people living with dementia meaningful opportunities to make things that are of, and for, 'the moment' through spontaneity, group co-creation and improvisation.

To date, there has been a wide body of research that has explored group-based creative activity for people living with dementia. While we can examine individual momentary experiences gained in this way, it may limit our understanding of the more everyday creative experiences, including the kind also known as 'little-c' creativity (Bellass et al. 2019). As an example, 'little-c' creativity might look like the creation of visual flashcards to support someone's daily routine or creating a scrapbook. In comparison, 'big C' creativity would be more in line with what we may think of as the creation of a visual masterpiece or composing a concerto.

Understanding everyday creativity might therefore mean paying close attention to the creative ways in which people with dementia live with their diagnosis in their day-to-day lives, such as through improvisation in the use of language or imaginative solutions for adapting their home environment to compensate for sensory deficits. However, group-based cultural or creative experiences, such as improvised music-making, appear to afford people living with dementia an opportunity to feel more connected to other people through a shared creative endeavour (Dowlen et al. 2021). Moreover, such benefits can also act as a springboard for the telling of individual life stories or act as a platform for reminiscence activities. In turn, this can enhance feelings of individual and collective well-being.

While there may be many benefits shared with other group-based leisure activities (e.g. football, gardening, cooking), it is the opportunity to create something together 'in the moment' that enables people living with dementia to express themselves in music, without the need for words, that interests. In the context of our own research focusing on live and spontaneous musical improvisation performed by people living with dementia, music afforded moments for sharing life story through musical improvisation where the sounds were used to spark a musical conversation and where words did not come so easily. The two of us writing this chapter felt strongly that we wanted to capture the lived experience of people with dementia participating in music; John has written about these 'in the moment' experiences for many years and Robyn has developed visual methodologies using video in this context. Through our separate and combined research, we have formed a strong collaborative relationship with Manchester Camerata (an orchestra and registered charity) over the past decade, and have conducted research alongside *Music in Mind*, Manchester Camerata's established music programme for people living with dementia. We draw on this research and partnership working in the 'case study' section of this chapter to emphasize the value of musical improvisation in the context of the lived experience of dementia. The improvisations we have observed in this work are initiated and sustained by people living with dementia truly 'in the moment' – only captured because the group formed the basis for a research case study. So, the question emerges, if we wish to create services that better support people living with dementia's well-being and everyday citizenship, how do we begin to evaluate and understand the value of these everyday leisurely 'moments' when they are often fleeting in time and may be difficult to capture?

Capturing the value of creative moments in research

As discussed earlier, the ways in which the creative arts have been framed and evaluated in research has largely been dominated by biomedical approaches to dementia. These will often involve measures being used before and after an intervention to assess its effect on a person's unmet needs, well-being or quality of life or qualitative methods that retrospectively examine lived experience. However, when we reduce creative experiences to this way of thinking, we are at risk of missing a wealth of information that might be available through taking a more momentary approach to understanding their value for people living with dementia. Such moments may also act to support and preserve the everyday citizenship of people living with dementia.

Telling the stories of people living with dementia as experienced through the creative arts is complex. As Basting (2020: 20) writes:

> Everyone has stories inside them; everyone has some kind of tool for expressing these stories; everyone has barriers keeping their stories from coming out – some more than others; it is up to us [as researchers, artists, carers etc.] to figure out how to invite the story out and how to listen it into existence.

Methodological development beyond traditional research methods and towards more creative approaches placing the voices of people living with dementia at their centre (Zeilig et al. 2014) provide ways to understand the everyday lived experiences of people with dementia. This is particularly important, given that some may not be able to express these verbally. Thus, creative participatory methods can help us as researchers to capture and share the stories of people living with dementia as they engage with creativity in their everyday lives.

As we shared earlier, while there has been a discussion about 'moments' and the 'here and now' for many years in the context of the creative arts and dementia (including through Dementia Care Mapping, for instance), there has been very little methodological innovation in this area that might allow researchers to unpick the idea of moments and how they contribute to the experiences of people living with dementia. However, Strohmaier et al. (2021), for example, have used the Canterbury Wellbeing Scales – a Visual Analogue Scale where measurements are taken in short intervals over the duration of an arts-based session across five subscales (happy/sad, well/unwell, interested/bored, confident/not confident and optimistic/not optimistic) – to capture 'in the moment' or short-term changes in well-being. Additionally, an example taken from the practice of co-developing textiles alongside people living with dementia includes the use of embodied and sensory methods (Fleetwood-Smith et al. 2022), but while this approach may allow for the examination of the momentary, it is time intensive and requires the researcher to embed themselves within the world as lived and experienced by people living with dementia. Such an immersive approach to research also requires a high degree of researcher reflexivity and understanding of the complex ethical nuances that can occur in these moments.

Basting (2020: 119) alludes to the idea that moments can be held as memories by those who support people living with dementia when she writes:

> Will Mr Wilson remember the moment? We can't know. But Elaine, Sheila, Bruce and I [the facilitators] know that we will and, holding that memory for him, we can invite him back to that memory again and again.

This quote brings us to a consideration of John's descriptions of sequential and cyclical continuum of moments, namely: creating – being (in) – ending – reliving the moment (Keady et al. 2022). In such an approach, there is an opportunity for the findings of the research process to 'invite' people living with dementia back into their creative experience and to relive the moment once again. To illustrate, we have found that data elicitation methods (i.e. the use of photo, video, objects etc. in prompting conversation) are particularly powerful within this context. Such methods also help people living with dementia to overcome some of the communication challenges associated with the condition, as well as giving them clear agency within the research process (Nedlund et al. 2019). There is also a role in these creative social research methods for family carers, creative arts facilitators and those supporting people living with dementia in a professional capacity, to interpret the multiple layers of experience held within the moment and reflect on the moment as part of the trajectory of each person's life story.

In the next section we present a case study showing how video-elicitation methods were used to understand the lived experiences of people living with dementia taking part in an improvisation-based music-making programme. While this was a pre-planned, time-limited (15-week) music programme, such methods could be applied more broadly by researchers and art practitioners to understand how people living with dementia experience leisure and leisure time. This section is written in the first person from the perspective of Robyn, who conducted her doctoral work within this setting.

Case study: Music in Mind

Overview

Manchester Camerata is a chamber orchestra based in the city of Manchester (UK). Its *Music in Mind* programme is for people living with dementia and their family carers, or those supporting them in a professional capacity. The same group members attend each week to ensure space for musical development as well as the opportunity to develop connections with each other. The programme has been delivered in community settings, day care centres, care homes, housing schemes and hospital wards. It is cofacilitated by a music therapist and a Manchester Camerata musician, combining therefore the skills of the therapist and that of a professional musician. This principle of cofacilitation enables a music-making space defined by creativity and leisure, rather than specific therapeutic outcomes alone.

The principles of *Music in Mind* afford a context where the person living with dementia is given choice and the opportunity to be creative. Musical improvisations, using tuned and untuned percussive instruments as well as the person's own vocalizations, are supported by the musicians, enabling the person living with dementia to situate themselves in a supportive music-making environment where their musical contributions are heard, responded to and valued. The aim, therefore, is not to look for any reduction in unmet need, but, rather, to support all the participants to explore the different musical instruments, to have fun with others in a light-hearted environment and – importantly – to feel listened to.

Within my research I aimed to develop a thematic description of the 'in the moment' embodied and sensory experiences of people living with dementia when they engage with music and the *Music in Mind* programme. To build a context for this ambition, we reviewed the qualitative literature that sought to understand the benefits of music for people living with dementia (Dowlen et al. 2018). Through this process we found that, although a wide range of benefits were reported (including feeling connected to oneself and others; affirming the person's sense of identity; developing new skills etc.), there was a strong reliance on traditional qualitative research methods such as interviews and focus groups. These limited the inclusion of people living with dementia in the research process, leaving only the voices of those who had the capacity to consent to be heard. I therefore began to explore different and more creative social research methods. More importantly, I wanted to explore methods that centred the creativity of people living with dementia taking part in the programme.

Methods for the momentary

Research into the experiences of people living with dementia and their family carers has observed the value of sensory and visual methods for understanding the everyday experiences of people living with dementia during, for example, hairdressing or care tasks (Ward et al. 2016). Visual methods are considered particularly important for dementia studies as they can allow people living with dementia to actively engage in the research process without the need to rely on verbal communication skills. Video is one of those methods used to explore the everyday and momentary experiences of people living with dementia. Using it in the *Music in Mind* case study, a combination of video observation and video-elicitation interviews enabled the in-depth exploration of 'in the moment' experience. Video provided a permanent record of the music sessions that could be reviewed outside of the field setting moment by moment with people living with dementia.

During one *Music in Mind* programme (15 sessions), I situated myself with three video cameras to explore the experiences of six people living with dementia, and four family carers. Two cameras were fixed, recording the two hemispheres of the circle, and capturing interactions that occurred in its centre. I operated the third camera by hand to capture more detail relating to facial expression and embodied gestures. Instead of sitting on the extremities of the circle as an 'outside' observer, I actively took part in the *Music in Mind* sessions through playing instruments and singing with the group. This enabled the development of a stronger rapport between group members and myself.

The value of recording the musical atmosphere created and experienced by people living with dementia within the context of *Music in Mind* was twofold. Firstly, it provided an opportunity for me to return to 'the moment' time and time again outside of the context of the sessions, to interpret the 'in the moment' embodied and sensory experiences of people living with dementia. Secondly, it provided video that could be used to help people living with dementia 'relive' the moment through video-elicitation interviews. This provided an additional layer of interpretation by people living with dementia and their family carers, giving greater depth and validation to the findings.

In between the *Music in Mind* sessions, participants were invited to take part in video-elicitation interviews within their own homes as individuals or as a couple. The primary purpose of these interviews was to enable participants to return to 'the moment' using video as a prompt and basis for reflective discussion. For example, singing familiar melodies from the *Music in Mind* sessions signalled a recognition of the songs outside the music-making space. It also highlighted the need to consider the data generated in the interview beyond spoken words (e.g. pointing, foot tapping, smiling and laughing). As there were a wide range of communication abilities and styles represented within the group, video provided a platform for discussion which elicited a greater response from people living with dementia than may have been afforded by a traditional semi-structured interview alone. This observation, echoed within the wider literature which uses video-elicitation interviews, strengthens the case for using the method in populations who may face difficulties when engaging with more traditional qualitative methods.

Using this combination of visual methods showed us that each person living with dementia had a unique experience held within these musical moments. This further highlighted the incomplete picture that is gained when only using pre/post approaches to understand the value of the creative arts. We were able to use the video data and the interview transcripts to build individual case studies of each person living with dementia as a musician, rather than 'patient' in need of 'therapeutic intervention'. These case studies presented the improvisations that were created and sustained by people living with dementia and showed how musical improvisation allowed each person to bring elements of their life story to the forefront (Dowlen et al. 2021). An illustrative case example is presented at the end of this section.

While the person living with dementia may not have remembered the sharing of their life story each week, the facilitating musicians held these memories for them and reintroduced them at poignant moments across the 15 weeks. Building on the point made by Basting quoted earlier, this highlights the role that can be played by others in holding moments for people living with dementia so that their stories can be told even when they do not have the words to express them. This holding of moments is not limited to researchers or artists such as musicians; indeed, family carers and formal carers hold these stories and memories within their everyday lives. Perhaps the creative arts can provide further opportunities to connect with people living with dementia in a more fun, spontaneous and meaningful way?

Case example: Mary

In this case example, we introduce Mary (a pseudonym) and share some of her interactions with music during the *Music in Mind* sessions. We reflect on how the visual methods enabled us to build a holistic and warm understanding of Mary's life story, and the way music interacted with her spirituality both within and beyond sessions. This is only a glimpse of Mary's story in the context of *Music in Mind* – a fuller account can be found in Dowlen (2019).

Mary had moved to Manchester from her home country of Nigeria in the early 2000s to work as a nurse. She was diagnosed with young onset Alzheimer's disease in 2013 and had found it difficult to come to terms with her diagnosis, leading her to experience depression and withdrawing from her social networks (especially her church community). She had felt as if her friends and her church had deserted her because of her diagnosis, and did not see a future for herself, as she recounted in one of our interviews: 'All I could remember was just to cover my nakedness and sit there waiting for the day I will die. I will sit down, I will be thinking of which music will be best for me when I am dead and how will I arrange for my funeral.'

Mary had no formal musical training but engaged with music when attending church, having been a part of several church choirs during her lifetime. She made it clear to me that her favourite music was gospel and worship music. Mary held very strong beliefs about the role that music had played in helping her to overcome the depression she had experienced and believed 'God' was working through the *Music in Mind* musicians, project team and group members to help her through a difficult point in her life. This came out during our video-elicitation interviews together, where seeing the group members in the video led to Mary recounting her feelings of connection to the group: 'Believing in God and believing in the people I'm working with that are looking at me, trusting that God is using them to heal me. God can come from heaven, but can pass through people to get to you and reach.'

Mary saw *Music in Mind* as an extension of her personal worship. She would attend sessions dressed in beautiful traditional Nigerian outfits, which she had made herself as a skilled seamstress. It was clear she saw music-making as a serious part of her leisure and dressed in her finest clothing when attending the sessions. Mary also used religious music within the sessions as a means of evangelizing to the group and introduced the melody for 'Oh When the Saints' in week five of the programme. This melody became a motif for Mary, with her introducing it in most sessions. During the weeks when Mary was not in attendance in the session, the musicians would introduce the melody into the group enabling Mary's presence to be felt by the group, even though she was not physically there.

We wanted to understand Mary's intentions behind introducing this specific melody into the group. The following excerpt from our second video-elicitation interview highlights Mary's motives for introducing the familiar melody into the group week after week:

Robyn: So when you sing it with the group, is it, do you start it because you want everyone…

Mary: To go to heaven. No I don't want anybody left out. Everybody like us, we are happy. I want us to meet there and say, 'Oh, so you made it to heaven. Oh Mary, you made it to heaven. Phillip [another group member] you made it to heaven.' … I know the saints have somewhere to go and I want the group to go there. That is why sometimes at the end; before we say [sings] 'Goodbye', I will sing that one. If we don't meet next Wednesday, by chance, if anybody were to die, we march to heaven.

This quote showcases the value Mary placed on music as a connector not only in this life, but to her vision of her life after death. Her spontaneous introduction of 'Oh When the Saints', in that moment in week five, illuminated her desire to stay connected to the group both within and outside the weekly sessions and formed an extension to her spirituality.

A moments-focused approach therefore enabled a deeper understanding of the role and value of music in Mary's life, and how it enabled her to feel connected and supported during a challenging point in her life. The focus on 'the moment' allowed Mary to be connected to the group spiritually, emotionally and physically within and beyond the sessions. Mary scheduled her whole week around *Music in Mind*, making sure that she had no conflicting appointments or going along to parts of the session before attending medical appointments. She did not want to miss out on these opportunities for connection afforded through making music with the group. It was clear through our interactions with Mary that music had been a source of comfort throughout her life, especially in the context of her church. Her diagnosis of dementia, however, led her to feel disconnected from and deserted by the church – the place where she had had consistent musical experiences across her lifetime. *Music in Mind* created the option for Mary to envisage her own community where her diagnosis was unimportant – a place she could connect to herself, her community and her God.

Finding meaning in moments

While there are many opportunities and benefits afforded through time-limited creative arts 'interventions', in this chapter we have shown how framing these experiences as purely 'therapeutic' may reduce our view of the experiences of people living with dementia to a focus on addressing their unmet needs. This framing has also led to a lack of understanding of the role the creative arts play as leisure activities across a person's whole life-course (including before dementia), and about how meaning can be created in the everyday lives of people living with dementia above and beyond care-based tasks. It is evident that people living with dementia are often not given a choice over when and how they engage with everyday creativity, with there being more emphasis placed on providing group-based scheduled activity. Realizing these often fleeting creative moments can be challenging for researchers, but as we have seen in this chapter, methodological innovation using visual and video methods appears to be making headway in capturing moments and supporting people living with dementia to relive them once again.

So what does this mean in practice?

For those supporting or enabling the involvement in leisure of people living with dementia

- Framing creative arts as leisure activities that are part of everyday life opens opportunities for engagement in the everyday, rather than purely as 'interventions' at times of need.
- Fashion as many opportunities as possible for people living with dementia to participate in creative leisure activity.
- Gather information about people living with dementia's life stories to create meaningful opportunities for participation and interaction.
- Recognize that everyone's experience of an activity will be personal to them.
- Take photos and video films and recordings of activity (with permission) to help the person living with dementia to recall and relive the positive memories and experiences after the event.

For people living with dementia or their informal or family carers

- Taking part in a creative activity can be a great way of enjoying time 'in the moment'. It can increase the person's sense of well-being and creates opportunities to have fun with other people. All those involved can decide how much they want to contribute, and at their own pace.
- It is sometimes difficult to tell beforehand whether someone is going to enjoy a particular activity or not. No one should be made to go again to a group they do not like.

- Photos and video films and recordings of activity can help people enjoy recalling and reliving positive memories and experiences after the event.

For researchers

- Framing the creative arts as leisure activities rather than inherently 'therapeutic' activity requires the development of innovative methods to capture the experience of those living with dementia.
- Researchers should be open to learning and undertaking new ways of 'doing' research that does not rely on capturing the person living with dementia's spoken word.
- We have found visual and sensory methods to be particularly helpful in this context and can support people living with dementia to 'relive' significant moments with researchers.
- The voices of people living with dementia need to be prioritized further within this area – in particular, understanding how the creative arts have intersected with their life stories and how their embodied selfhood is showcased through creative and improvised moments.

References

Bamford, C. and Bruce, E. (2000) Defining the outcomes of community care: The perspectives of older people with dementia and their carers, *Ageing & Society*, 20(5): 543–70.

Basting, A. (2020) *Creative Care: A Revolutionary Approach to Dementia and Elder Care*. New York: HarperCollins.

Bellass, S., Balmer, A., May, V. et al. (2019) Broadening the debate on creativity and dementia: A critical approach, *Dementia*, 18(7–8): 2799–820.

Bryden, C. (1998) *Who Will I Be When I Die?* London: Jessica Kingsley Publishers.

Bryden, C. (2005) *Dancing with Dementia: My Story of Living Positively with Dementia*. London: Jessica Kingsley Publishers.

Dowlen, R. (2019) The 'in the moment' musical experiences of people with dementia: A multiple-case study approach. PhD thesis, University of Manchester.

Dowlen, R., Keady, J., Milligan, C. et al. (2018) The personal benefits of musicking for people living with dementia: A thematic synthesis of the qualitative literature, *Arts & Health*, 10(3): 197–212.

Dowlen, R., Keady, K., Milligan, C. et al. (2021) In the moment with music: An exploration of the embodied and sensory experiences of people living with dementia during improvised music making, *Ageing and Society*, 42(11): 2642–64.

Fleetwood-Smith, R., Tischler, V. and Robson, D. (2022) Using creative, sensory and embodied research methods when working with people with dementia: A method story, *Arts & Health*, 14(3): 263–79.

Keady, J.D., Campbell, S., Clark, A. et al. (2022) Re-thinking and re-positioning 'being in the moment' within a continuum of moments: Introducing a new conceptual framework for dementia studies, *Ageing & Society*, 42(3): 681–702.

Mason, J. (2018) *Affinities: Potent Connections in Personal Life*. Cambridge: Polity Press.

Nedlund, A-C., Bartlett, R. and Clarke, C.L. (2019) *Everyday Citizenship and People with Dementia*. London: Dunedin.

Smith, L., Phillipson, L. and Knight, P. (2021) Re-imagining care transitions for people with dementia and complex support needs in residential aged care: Using co-designed sensory objects and a focused ethnography to recognise micro transitions, *Ageing & Society*, 43(1): 1–23.

Strohmaier, S., Homans, K.M., Hulbert, S. et al. (2021) Arts-based interventions for people living with dementia: Measuring 'in the moment' wellbeing with the Canterbury Wellbeing Scales, *Wellcome Open Research*, 6: 59.

Swaffer, K. (2015) Dementia and prescribed disengagement™, *Dementia*, 14(1): 3–6.

Ward, M.C., Milligan, C., Rose, E., Elliot, M. et al. (2021) The benefits of community-based participatory arts activities for people living with dementia: A thematic scoping review, *Arts & Health*, 13(3): 213–39.

Ward, R., Campbell, S. and Keady, J. (2016) 'Gonna make yer gorgeous': Everyday resistance and transformation in the care-based hair salon, *Dementia*, 15(3): 395–413.

Zeilig, H., Killick, J. and Fox, C. (2014) The participative arts for people living with a dementia: A critical review, *International Journal of Ageing and Later Life*, 9(1): 7–34.

7 Sport and physical activity

Chris Russell

Summary

The benefits to physical health for individuals taking part in sport and physical activity are well known. Spending time with others while participating can help people feel happier in themselves and with life in general. People living with dementia should expect to benefit from sport and physical activity just like anyone else. There is research which reports on the physical benefits for people living with dementia. However, less is known about how taking part might influence the experience of everyday life of people living with dementia, and how individuals may feel about themselves and their continued place in the world as a result. In this chapter we take a closer look at the experiences of some people living with dementia regularly taking part in sport and physical activity. For example, activities include playing badminton, swimming or going to the gym in their local leisure centre. We examine what it might mean for people living with dementia taking part as they go about their everyday lives. This is helpful in moving us on from thinking about dementia as purely a medical condition. If individuals are able to choose what they do and how they do it, sport and physical activity can strengthen the feeling that they are keeping a place in the world. For example, this feeling can be enhanced because people are learning new skills, doing things that are enjoyable and being with others in ways that feel pleasant. The chapter sets out recommendations for those wishing to offer physical activity to people living with dementia as part of everyday life. These include tailoring what they do to support individual participants living with dementia, building relationships with and between people living with dementia as they participate, offering choice in what activities are available and using a diversity of physical spaces flexibly to maximize the ability of people to participate in a manner that is enjoyable.

Setting the scene: physical activity and dementia

Interest in sport and physical activity for people living with dementia has grown, particularly in relation to preventing dementia, the role sport might have played in causing dementia, and in sports reminiscence. There is an indication, for example, that for some people, participation in physical activity can be beneficial in preventing dementia or delaying symptoms. However, this is a complex area, and the evidence is mixed (Liu-Ambrose et al. 2018). There is also increasing concern about links between head injuries and dementia. This has potential consequences for sports such as rugby, boxing and football, where impact to the head of participants can contribute to the emergence of symptoms related to dementia-causing illnesses for some people playing those sports (Stewart 2021). Sports reminiscence, meanwhile, has been employed over many years with people living with dementia. It has had several aims, ranging from aspiring to hold a therapeutic function to providing opportunities for social contact.

An area that has been less explored, however, is the opportunity for people living with dementia to engage in physical activity, as they wish – in other words, physical activity available as a leisure choice for people living with dementia. Engaging in physical activity should be a right and a potential pleasure for everyone, if this is what they choose to do with their time. It is an indictment that this has not been something that people living with dementia can take for granted.

What participation in physical activity might mean for individuals within their everyday lives is not well understood. Exploring the experiences of people living with dementia contributes to moving us on from thinking about dementia as purely a medical condition. There are examples of how things are changing, with sports clubs and providers of physical activity becoming increasingly keen to offer opportunities to people living with dementia (for example, the walking football offered at Hampden Park Scotland, described later in this book – see Chapter 13). This chapter explains the ideas and theory underpinning this change, setting out ways in which such progression should happen, with the provision of physical activity as its focus.

Findings from a UK research study that set out to deepen understanding about the role of sport in people's lives provide the foundations for the chapter. I completed this research with four people living with dementia who engaged regularly in physical activity such as playing badminton, swimming or going to the gym over a 12-month period, at their local Leisure and Fitness Centres, or Centres.[1] I also interviewed members of their families and sports professionals (referred to as Workers) over the same period. Theories are offered to support the discussion. For example, an understanding of *well-being* as it has been applied to the leisure context, *casual and serious leisure* – which assist comprehension of the motivation of participants living with dementia to engage in physical activity, and *opportunity structures* – which help draw the learning set out in this chapter together.

Physical activity as a leisure choice for people living with dementia

The person and the social context for their participation

This research was informed by person-centred principles and values underpinning social citizenship. The focus was on the four people living with dementia who were the participants in the research, along with those who engaged in activity alongside them. Pseudonyms are used throughout.

Jacqui was 63 years old at the time of the research. Physical activity had been of some importance to her, on and off, throughout her life. Since she had retired on grounds of ill health caused by dementia, Jacqui had attended her local Centre regularly. She enjoyed exercise classes and walks organized by Patrick, a Worker at the Centre. Jacqui was diagnosed with dementia with Lewy bodies, meaning she had difficulty with posture and physical dexterity, alongside compromised ability to read and write. Jacqui also had minor hallucinations which hindered her ability to orientate herself to her surroundings and caused some short-term memory loss. Living alone, Jacqui attended the Centre solo.

Paul was 79 years of age. Sport played a fundamental part in his life. He had been a cricketer and footballer, playing for his local amateur teams. He now participated in leisure alongside his wife Connie at the Centre close to where he lived, where Martin and Jane were the Workers supporting this activity. Paul was diagnosed with Alzheimer's disease two years before the research began. Symptoms included short-term memory loss and anxiety (possibly as a result). He had lost confidence in being able to follow his train of thought, and this impeded his willingness to speak in public. Paul had difficulty remembering details about recent events but retained the ability to recall things that happened longer ago.

Ivan was 64 years old at the time the research commenced. He had always played sport and engaged in physical activity. In earlier years that had included cricket and football. Latterly, he attended his local Centre where he took part, often alongside his wife Jemma, in fitness classes and gym sessions. He was supported by a Worker, Kyle. Ivan had been diagnosed at the age of 57 with corticobasal degeneration, a rare form of dementia-causing illness, which resulted in increasing difficulty with speech, movement and dexterity. Ivan remained able to remember events, but struggled to articulate them verbally.

Leonard was 59 years old. He had disliked sport in his earlier life and only came to it in the years after his diagnosis, regularly attending alongside his wife, Caroline, at a Centre close to where the couple lived (the same one as Paul and Connie). Leonard enjoyed playing badminton and swimming. He had been diagnosed with posterior cortical atrophy three years before. This is a form of dementia-causing illness resulting in compromised visual ability and spatial judgement, as well as having an impact on short-term memory. Leonard had little difficulty with speech, though he occasionally felt muddled, struggling to find words as swiftly as he would have liked.

The perspectives and circumstances of individuals matter, but so do the broader features influencing everyday life – for example, the gender, ethnicity, sexuality and economic situation of participants in physical activity – as emphasized in the opening chapter of this book. An example highlighted in this research was the diversity of age of people living with dementia. Caroline raised a concern: 'It doesn't help that there's very little out there for young people with dementia.'

The point at which dementia enters a person's life will have implications for how that individual and those close to them view the future (Draper and Withall 2016), influencing in turn how they feel about physical activity and what part it might play in everyday life. Three of the participants in the research were aged under 70, and thus a lack of opportunity for support for younger people was keenly felt. However, all ages and abilities must have opportunities, and physical activity must be tailored in different ways to suit the needs and aspirations of individuals.

People living with dementia may also feel a sense of stigma, simply because of their diagnosis (Fletcher 2021). How people perceive their involvement in physical activity, especially if this is in a public setting, is thus important. Talking about how she and Paul felt about taking part in physical activity at their local Centre, Connie said: 'It's like people. You're not made to feel embarrassed or anything like that.' Thus, in this couple's case, the attitudes of others with whom they participated affected how comfortable they felt about their own engagement.

The domestic situation of individuals living with dementia, particularly if there are care partners or family carers involved, will influence the experience a person has of physical activity. For example, care partners and family carers will hold different perspectives to the person living with dementia, as their daily experiences will be different. The ability of family members who are care partners to sustain their own interests and wider acquaintances can be corroded by dementia (Clarke and Bailey 2016) because of the impact dementia has on the person they support. The situation of people with dementia living alone is less often considered and this has adverse consequences for the availability of support for individuals living in such circumstances (Bartlett 2022). Jacqui's accounts throughout this chapter are useful in remedying this.

There are other factors relating to individuals' experiences of dementia, highlighted by my research, that contribute to the context for their engagement in physical activity – for example, the symptoms of dementia and the part the person perceives these as playing in their life. As Jacqui said: 'It would be too easy not to do all this. Since I have been deteriorating it is an effort to do it.'

A person's experiences of engagement in physical activity may be influenced by health concerns beyond the symptoms of dementia. For example, here Caroline is discussing Leonard's difficulties with hearing linked to his earlier employment: 'He's got industrial deafness … when he was younger they didn't have health and safety issues around wearing ear defenders.'

Such difficulties with physical health may not be easy to recognize but must be anticipated. This is because sensory difficulties, such as sight or hearing loss, can exacerbate the sense of exclusion from everyday life a person living with dementia feels, compounding their isolation (Leroi 2020).

People living with dementia can support their sense of identity while taking part in physical activity through communication that uses the body (Wright 2018). Examples offered by participants in the research illuminate the importance of tailoring how physical activity is provided, and of including communication which does not rely on speech. For instance, Leonard showed how important this was to him when he said: 'I'm not so keen on table tennis. Cos, you can't really whack it can you? [laughing heartily] I think it's a bit of getting rid of aggression.'

This is an example of 'embodied identity mobility' – i.e. how identity can be shaped by individuals via intense use of their body in exercise. It has been argued that it is a way in which voices of people marginalized within society can be articulated (Mayoh et al. 2020).

Another example of the way in which non-verbal communication matters was noted by Jacqui: 'I only go by watching them, other people around me … On the whole I have to 'mirror'. Do what they are doing [the facilitator]. Not what they are saying. You need landmarks you can follow. Words are not directions to my short circuits.'

For Jacqui, watching the facilitator of the exercise class she was attending and copying his actions was more helpful than instruction given verbally. However, with potential sensory difficulties of the sort discussed above in mind, it is important to note that background noise and loud music may be a distraction to certain individuals.

People living with dementia will have different reasons for choosing to participate in physical activity. For some it will be about happiness and living a life of quality, which could be described as well-being. There are many definitions of well-being. An interpretation that is helpful with the subject matter of this chapter in mind is that offered by Mayoh and Jones (2015), because it illuminates several of its key themes. For example, the authors argue well-being for individuals is characterized by a sense of agency and situated freedom. Agency is being in control and feeling in control of what happens to you. Situated freedom is where individuals continue to engage with the world and social contexts – for example, obligations towards others – while at the same time retaining the opportunity and ability to exercise free will and choice. Mayoh and Jones (2015: 243) go on to describe 'spatial dwelling-mobility' where well-being is fostered for individuals through engagement within familiar and comforting environments, alongside opportunities for experiences presented via sporting activity.

Jemma explained how the reasons Ivan chose to participate were linked to well-being when she said: 'He just likes the feeling of getting hot and sweaty in sport … to feel you've had a workout, and come off thinking I feel so much better for that.' This mirrored what Mayoh and Jones had said about individuals valuing agency and situated freedom.

Individuals may feel motivated to engage in physical activity because they wish to learn new skills, sustain the abilities they have or engage in a way that feels meaningful. Theoretical understandings of leisure can assist here – for example, 'casual' and 'serious' leisure, concepts explained by Stebbins in the foreword to the book.

People living with dementia may wish to engage in physical activity as casual leisure, as part of the 'everyday', which is so important in realizing social citizenship for individuals (Bartlett and O'Connor 2007, 2010). For example, Leonard recounted a reason he enjoyed games of badminton, where he felt able to play with freedom and vigour: 'There are no rules!'

Figure 7.1 People living with dementia will wish to participate in physical activity for many reasons, just as anyone would

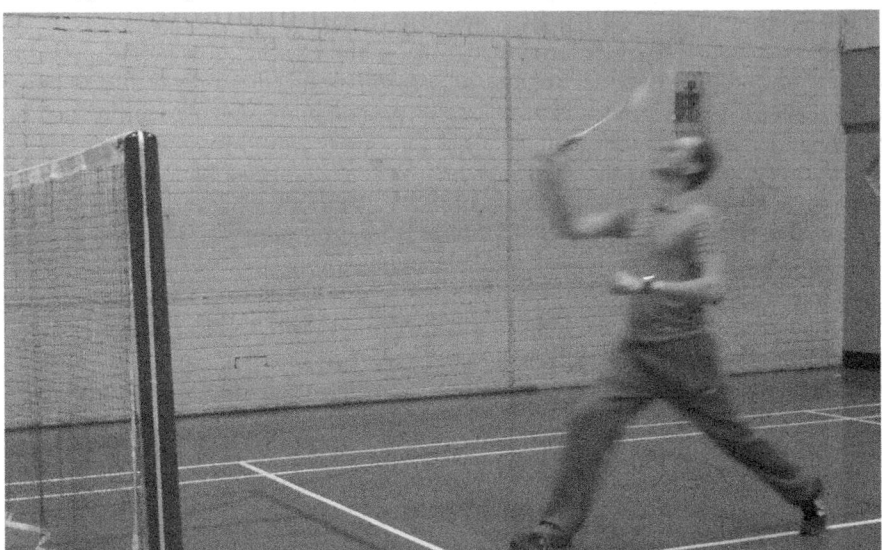

Just like anyone else, however, people living with dementia may hold contrasting motivations for engagement in physical activity. Thus, serious leisure can play a part in motivation too, as the following accounts illustrate. Here, for example, Jacqui explains her reasons for participating: 'I want to push it, that I feel the benefit of it. And in a day or two if I don't continue I know that I will feel it.' Later she added: 'I want to keep my … stamina, and I hope that I can keep pushing myself to do something to keep my strength up as much as I can, and my talents don't lie in anything else.' This illustrates serious leisure, demonstrating how Jacqui wishes to feel after engaging in physical activity. The everyday for Jacqui relates to having aspiration and choice as part of her participation.

Paul offered some of his reasons for continuing to engage in physical activity: 'You win some and you lose some, but you always try your best.' Then, with a smile on his face, he added the following, during a break from a game of table tennis: 'You never lose it!' Paul's dementia was relatively advanced. Physically well, he was experiencing challenges to his cognitive ability. His example shows, however, that elements of serious leisure can apply for individuals at later stages of their illness.

Motivation for participation in physical activity can vary; this acts as a reminder of the necessity to sustain a person-centred approach, because people might want to do different things on different days for different reasons.

For example, in the earlier instance Leonard had indicated his motivation was linked to casual leisure. However, another time he reflected on the reasons he chose to engage in more vigorous physical activity: 'It got me breathing. Got a bit of a sweat on… [laughing…] you feel you have done something … being physically fit, being able to do what I want to be able to do.' Leonard was keen to participate in ways that were substantial and fulfilling, and where new experiences were gained and put into action. He went on to link his motivation to losses in life caused by dementia: 'You've got to find something else to do and you don't know what that's going to be and whether you can do it or not.'

Engaging in physical activity offered Leonard purpose. It was something he could do and had control over. He valued this, as he went on to say, 'you're achieving something … actually doing something physically … being there and doing it … Brilliant, great … love it'.

Individuals living with dementia commonly experience feelings of loss, particularly of ability and sense of status within daily life (Sharp 2019). Aspects of Leonard and Jacqui's accounts have alluded to this. Loss might be caused by the symptoms of dementia illnesses and/or the reactions of others towards people living with dementia. Participants in the research showed how engaging in serious leisure could help them assuage loss and look forward instead to novel experiences and use of new skills. While this will not be the case for everyone, loss should not be accepted as inevitable, and engagement in physical activity is one way in which this can be challenged by individuals and those supporting them.

The spaces within which physical activity takes place

The 'where' of the physical spaces of leisure must not be separated from the 'how' of engagement with physical activity for people living with dementia. This is because spaces influence the quality of experience through an impact on feelings of well-being and a sense of place in the world held by participants living with dementia (Clarke and Bailey 2016).

Spaces offered for the pursuit of physical activity must be accessible to people living with dementia. For example, undue distance to the venue and problems with ease of access can hinder the ability to exercise social citizenship, as Jacqui explained while outlining practical difficulties with attending the Centre: 'I don't like not living so near, it limits when I come … it is the cost of petrol. The public transport is difficult, you need to know what goes where and when.'

Jacqui also identified aspects of the layout of the space influencing her experience of engaging in physical activity: 'I have to go by the same routine. Which sounds silly. The same cubicle, the same locker, and that's another automatic pilot cos something new is strange.' Other aspects of the layout of space can affect quality of experience. For example, the environment and ambience of the space mattered. A compressed space felt crowded and difficult to access. For example, Jacqui highlighted things she disliked about the gym: 'It's all … crowded into you and it's not so easy to, to just walk in and do.' This hindered her motivation and ability to exercise. Far better for her was the larger and more open space of the sports hall, where she could engage in physical activity such as light exercise classes, alongside others. This was where Jacqui found socializing easier. She said: 'You can get together and talk ... You wouldn't do that in a gym ... you're not getting any interaction ... It is relaxed. You can come and go. You don't feel threatened.'

Connie confirmed the positive effect spaces can have, her account highlighting the good feeling contact with everyday daily life induced. It was the mix of people and ages using the Centre space where she and Paul took part in physical activity: 'It's a nice meeting place, very social ... You get all sorts of age groups coming in ... the children that go swimming, and all the mums and babies, and the fitness classes, there's all sorts going on ... Nice to see a few friendly faces when you walk in.'

Spaces for physical activity do not have to be indoors. Here, for example, Jacqui comments on the imaginative and creative use of space outside the walls of the Centre as a venue for an organized walk she regularly took part in:

> It's nice to get outside ... you can see sunshine, the trees, the gardens and hear the birds ... I enjoy this time. It feels like hard work and that is satisfying, but it helps me destress too. I feel like I have really done something. Then I can go home and rest ... [it's] a good way to lose yourself. It's good to chat.

The walk is attractive for several reasons. It enables Jacqui to push and test herself, it is part of the broad choice of physical activity on offer (more on this below), it provides the chance of company and it also makes positive use of outdoor spaces.

The opportunity to participate in physical activity

We move on to consider approaches that can facilitate physical activity for people living with dementia.

Personhood is understood as the relationships an individual living with dementia has with others, and their quality in terms of sustaining feelings of self and identity (Kitwood and Brooker 2019; Brooker and Latham 2016). Thus, people offering physical activity are encouraged to build relationships with people living with dementia as they participate. Jacqui confirmed the significance of this when discussing Patrick's approach: 'He's always there for a chat ... he always asks after you and everyone.'

Jacqui emphasizes how the approach to facilitation extends beyond the activity itself. 'He's a friendly kind of ... characteristics, and he obviously has known us from day one. He's the one that signed us up. So he's seen the progress up or down or static that we've made.'

The feeling generated, built upon personhood, enables Jacqui to sustain her place in the world. Through her account she has summarized some of the essentials to good facilitation: being friendly, being interested in her as a participant and knowing her for long enough to have a sense of how she is in relation to the progression of dementia.

Leonard's experience of Martin's approach was similarly illustrative: 'He's always around, and he's always helpful … You can ask him any questions that you want to.' This relationship had been built from the first point Leonard and Caroline had engaged in physical activity at the Centre, highlighting the importance of the welcome individuals living with dementia receive. Caroline related how it was the proactive approach to the welcome and its genuine feel that counted. For example, she described what worked for her and Leonard, and the ways Jane and Martin both contributed: 'The fact that they're very welcoming so there's nobody new that arrives … that doesn't immediately feel part of the group … When we first arrived … Jane immediately came out and welcomed us in, and Martin then came along straight away.' Connie, who attended the same Centre alongside Paul, confirmed the positive nature of this approach, saying: 'It was very welcoming. Jane said, "It's your first time, you're new … Oh I'll sit you by Anne and Mick", who was a lady and her husband who'd been coming since its [the group's] inception … they were very nice.'

Figure 7.2 Facilitation of physical activity is multifaceted. Priorities include promoting personhood and collaboration with and alongside participants.

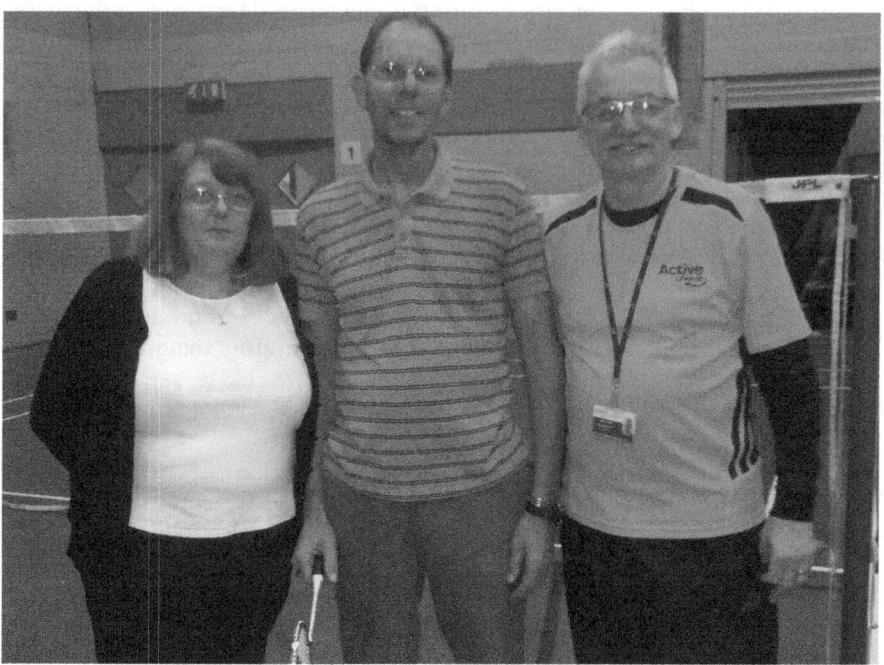

However, building relationships must extend beyond the level of the Worker to individual participants. Facilitators should encourage and support opportunities for people living with dementia to be sociable, because this enhances the value participants feel about their involvement. For example Jacqui related: 'There's two or three more ladies that have started using the gym and going to other sessions such as the get-together session ... the fact it's the social and getting to meet people ... that's quite a big thing.' Jacqui went on to confirm a significant reason for her enjoyment in attending: 'Cos of the people that are here, that I know.'

Leonard described how it was the contacts he established that made him want to attend the Centre. He explained how physical activity could contribute to this: 'It's not necessarily about beating the person. Winning isn't necessary. It's about having a good game. It's about enjoying playing together ... not winning, it's more being mutually competitive, that's what I like.'

Sharing the experience of playing a game was valued by Leonard. Reciprocity, the feeling of being with others and enjoying company, is a major factor in enabling people living with dementia to feel they retain an active place in the world (Kontos et al. 2017). Such experiences also provide examples of 'communicative leisure', as described by Spracklen (2013) – that is, leisure activity characterized by meaningfulness and self-affirmation for the person taking part. Leonard's reflections illustrate the opportunity physical activity provides for such constructive outcomes.

Workers can enable social citizenship to flourish through the opportunities they provide for physical activity. In turn this can be used by people living with dementia to influence additional aspects of their life, as Jacqui demonstrated when talking about getting to know others. Contacts made at the Centre led to trips out for meals, for example. Jacqui offered insight into how Workers can play a role enabling such relationships. For example, describing her experience of how Patrick facilitates the organized walk: 'He made sure that we're all a good group before we start.'

Reflecting on the priorities he holds for facilitation of physical activity, Martin explained it was about:

> The comradeship of it ... how they make ... friends ... a group ... It's like building a sort of network ... we offer a variety of different things, there's the singing, the sport, a chat, having a cup of tea ... we try to say...what else would you like to do? Get involved in the badminton ... go into the gym if you wish.

The proactive approach, witnessed at the point of the welcome, is repeated with effort to ascertain what people's preferences and aspirations are for their engagement in activity. This is accompanied with endeavour to find activities to meet these ambitions.

Caroline confirmed the approach when she recounted what Martin had said to her and Leonard at an early point in their participation in physical activity at the Centre: 'No you don't have to do singing, we can do this, we can do that. What else would you like to do? And [Martin] ... went into full gear to arrange a programme that would suit us.' In such ways, camaraderie and comradeship can be formed between and among participants.

Inherent in these accounts is having a choice about what activities individuals engage in, the range of activities on offer and the extent to which attendees choose to engage. For example, Jacqui related: 'The sport things are all here … I do odd bits of swimming … I do the walk and Thursday class … And I used to come to a Saturday group. And I helped out a lot.' Leonard corroborated this when he said he liked taking part because, 'There's lots I could do.'

Opportunities to engage in diverse activities can extend beyond participation, however, to include people living with dementia playing a role in facilitation. For example, Patrick related his experience of Jacqui's engagement in fitness classes: 'First person in, last person to go. Always will help me if I've set out equipment. She'll help me set it out, she'll help me put it away.'

Such examples highlight how agency is achieved through choice. Furthermore, people affected by dementia can also have the opportunity to influence how services are organized. Here, for example, Martin is commenting on his response to input from Leonard and Caroline in relation to the organization of public swimming at the Centre: 'I took that to the manager … and said … can [we] make those lanes bigger? So what they do now … at 12 o'clock … they'll put a double lane in.' This example, of a service receiving feedback, and using it to amend their offering, demonstrates how people living with dementia can realize social citizenship through their involvement in physical activity.

Facilitators must also retain awareness of the changing abilities that individuals living with dementia present. This returns to earlier discussions about well-being and to the priority for person-centred approaches. As an individual's ability to participate changes because of the progressive nature of dementia then alterations in attendance and participation will follow. This may feel uncomfortable for the person. For example, Jacqui said about her situation: 'I know a few years ago I was so fit, so able to do things, and now I fumble through.' She went on to provide additional perspective on life with dementia in the context of her experience in engagement in physical activity: 'It's funny because, because of my symptoms I'm worse off after three years, whereas the others are better.' Jacqui's account shows her awareness of the progressive nature of dementia and what this means. She is comparing her situation with other group members who are not living with dementia. Facilitators should consider the consequences for this in how activity is planned and delivered.

Physical activity will often be something happening in public, and by its nature demonstrate what might be construed as success or failure to the person taking part and to those around them. In these senses it is a transparent phenomenon. The possibility of what might feel like failure to a participant and its consequences should thus be anticipated by those facilitating physical activity to people living with dementia. Leonard offered an example, here linked to equipment he was using in the gym, on this occasion an exercise bike: 'The machine's moving for you … It seems to and I can't … get my feet to go into the same sort of rhythm as the bikes go … I got fed up with it, and so that was that … I just walked away.'

Leonard did not get on using the gym and its equipment and the outcome was extreme: he never used the gym again. Thus, it is a priority for services to offer facilitation and support so that people living with dementia can make the fullest use of equipment and opportunities related to physical activity.

Leonard's example highlights the broader risk that individuals might perceive failure as part of their engagement with physical activity. This can have a negative impact on participants, especially if individuals living with dementia already feel the sense of loss described earlier. Who do people have to seek comfort from if an instance of physical activity causes upset and despair? This question re-emphasizes the relational aspect to this area of everyday life. For example, the confidence to continue to engage, provided by the approach Patrick took to facilitation, was vital for Jacqui. Adjustment to life with dementia is fundamental to enabling individuals with the condition to live a life of quality (Brooker et al. 2017). Workers showed how what they did when they were alongside people living with dementia could support adjustment.

Risk is inherent to physical activity – risk of the type described above, where feelings of loss might be accentuated, and/or physical risk too (e.g. falls, pulled muscles). However, it is important to be sensible about risk (Department of Health 2010). Risk assessment must be reasonable and proportionate to take account of the individual's circumstances. Anyone participating in physical activity would expect to feel and to be as safe as possible. People living with dementia are no different, but it is wrong to limit opportunity based on presumptions made about dementia without considering the specific circumstances of the individual. Consider too the risk for individuals of *not* being enabled to do something. Being able to feel a sense of achievement is significant, providing opportunities for feelings of agency, and of sustaining a place in the world. For example, as he finished a game of badminton Leonard related: 'It takes your breath away. It's brilliant.'

Opportunity structures

As this chapter draws to a close, the theory of opportunity structures is offered to help bring learning together, and to illustrate how physical activity could be tailored to support adjustment to life with dementia for individuals. Opportunity structures is a theory whereby disabled participants use leisure and physical activity to reframe their identity to shape an ongoing sense of self, with sporting activities providing a context through which a stigmatized identity can be redefined by them (Lundberg et al. 2011).

Findings from the research showed that opportunity structures acted in combination with the life story and personal attributes of individuals living with dementia as they engaged at Centres, and the interaction those individuals had with others in Centre settings. Opportunity structures operated on the identity of participants in three ways, which sometimes overlapped. This was through:

- the physical activity itself (i.e. activities which enabled positive reformulation of identity, either through how participants felt about their engagement with them, or from feedback received from others)

- opportunity structures that helped people adjust to living with dementia (i.e. through Workers tailoring what they offered in ways to support people to be active citizens, to sustain participatory roles within the daily life of the Centre, and to organize what they did so people could recognize how engagement was having an impact on their perception of themselves)
- the diversity of activity available within Centres acting as opportunity structures (i.e. what was available within Centres helped people express their continuity of identity through the flexible and diverse nature of activities on offer – people living with dementia had a wide choice of what they wished to engage in).

The chance for people living with dementia to use leisure and physical activity to reframe their identity to shape an ongoing sense of self in the world is positive and powerful. Those planning to offer physical activity to people living with dementia are encouraged to note the influence opportunity structures can have in practice, when attention is also provided to the life story and personal attributes of participants.

So what does this mean in practice?

The chapter has focused on research and scholarship exploring how people living with dementia can participate in and enjoy physical activity as part of everyday life, if this is their wish. Implications derived from this are offered to inform practice.

For those supporting or enabling the involvement in leisure of people living with dementia

- A person-centred approach must infuse everything done by anyone with responsibility for the design and delivery of physical activity for people living with dementia. Examples provided include prioritizing getting to know participants well. People should have choice in what they do and how they go about it. Individuals should be offered the chance to learn new skills if this is their wish.
- Relationships are key. The concept of personhood is helpful by highlighting that it is by paying attention to how people are and can be alongside others that matters. Examples have emphasized how this must be a priority right from the moment of first welcome to an activity, and ever more afterwards. Spaces of leisure, their accessibility and how they are used can also contribute to fostering personhood and positive relationships.
- Physical activity has the potential to enable people living with dementia to sustain their place in the world. Involvement in physical activity can play a role in ensuring the social citizenship of individuals is maintained and strengthened, with the benefits that flow for a sense of well-being. Theories

of leisure – for example, causal and serious leisure and communicative leisure – can be incorporated into practice to strengthen the ability of physical activity to offer opportunities to people living with dementia to sustain their place in the world.

For people living with dementia or their informal or family carers

- The symptoms of dementia-causing illnesses change over time (because all dementias are progressive). Thus, what people living with dementia wish to do in terms of physical activity and how they go about it will also change as time passes.
- The layout and design of the spaces where physical activity takes place will influence the experience people have of participation, but so too will the extent that these spaces (or those close by) offer opportunity for social contact and socialization. What people need and require (in relation to both features) will alter over time.

Endnote

1   The definition of Leisure Centres (Centres) is based on the work of Taylor, Panagouleas and Ping Kung (2011). These are places situated within local neighbourhoods which are open to the public and provide a range of opportunities for physical activity and/or socialization. Typically, this will include the chance to take part in sport (for example badminton, table tennis, five-a-side-football etc.), physical activity in a gym or to use associated facilities such as a cafe/restaurant or communal meeting space. Provision may also include fitness classes or a swimming pool.

References

Bartlett, R. (2022) Inclusive (social) citizenship and persons with dementia, *Disability & Society*, 37(7): 1129–45.

Bartlett, R. and O'Connor, D. (2007) From personhood to citizenship: Broadening the lens for dementia practice and research, *Journal of Aging Studies*, 21(2): 107–18.

Bartlett, R. and O'Connor, D. (2010) *Broadening the Dementia Debate: Towards Social Citizenship*. Bristol: Policy Press.

Brooker, D., Evans, S.B. and Dröes, R.M. (2017) Framing outcomes of post-diagnostic psychosocial interventions in dementia, *Working with Older People*, 21(1): 13–21.

Brooker, D. and Latham, I. (2016) *Person-Centred Dementia Care: Making Services Better with the VIPS Framework*, 2nd edn. London and Philadelphia: Jessica Kingsley Publishers.

Clarke, C.L. and Bailey, C. (2016) Narrative citizenship, resilience and inclusion with dementia: On the inside or on the outside of physical and social places, *Dementia*, 15(3): 434–52.

Department of Health (2010) *'Nothing Ventured, Nothing Gained': Risk Guidance for Dementia*. London: DoH. Available at: https://assets.publishing.service.gov.uk/

government/uploads/system/uploads/attachment_data/file/215960/dh_121493.pdf (accessed 12 October 2021).

Draper, B. and Withall, A. (2016) Young onset dementia, *Internal Medicine Journal*, 46(7): 779–86.

Fletcher, J.R. (2021) Destigmatising dementia: The dangers of felt stigma and benevolent othering, *Dementia*, 20(2): 417–26.

Kitwood, T. and Brooker, D. (2019) *Dementia Reconsidered Revisited: The Person Still Comes First*. London: Open University Press.

Kontos, P., Miller, K.L. and Kontos, A.P. (2017) Relational citizenship: Supporting embodied selfhood and relationality in dementia care, *Sociology of Health and Illness*, 39(2): 182–98.

Leroi, I. (2020) 'Losing my glasses … losing my mind': Perspectives on sensory impairment, loneliness, social isolation and dementia, *International Journal of Geriatric Psychiatry*, 35(4): 335–7.

Liu-Ambrose, T., Barha, C.K. and Best, J.R. (2018) Physical activity for brain health in older adults, *Applied Physiology, Nutrition, and Metabolism*, 43(11): 1105–12.

Lundberg, N., Tanaguchi, S., McCormick, B. and Tibbs, C. (2011) Identity negotiating: Redefining stigmatized identities through adaptive sports and recreation participation among individuals with a disability, *Journal of Leisure Research*, 43(2): 205–25.

Mayoh, J. and Jones, I. (2015) Making well-being an experiential possibility: The role of sport, *Qualitative Research in Sport, Exercise and Health*, 7(2): 235–52.

Mayoh, J., Jones, I. and Prince, S. (2020) Women's experiences of embodied identity through active leisure, *Leisure Sciences*, 42(2): 170–84.

Sharp, B. (2019) Stress as experienced by people with dementia: An interpretative phenomenological analysis, *Dementia*, 18(4): 1427–45.

Spracklen, K. (2013) *Leisure, Sports and Society*. Basingstoke: Palgrave Macmillan.

Stewart, W. (2021) Sport associated dementia, *British Medical Journal*, 372: 168. DOI: 10.1136/bmj.n168.

Taylor, P., Panagouleas, T. and Ping Kung, S. (2011) Access to English public sector sports facilities by disadvantaged groups and the effect of financial objectives, *Managing Leisure*, 16(2): 128–41.

Wright, A. (2018) Exploring the relationship between community-based physical activity and wellbeing in people with dementia: A qualitative study, *Ageing and Society*, 38(3): 522–42.

8 Tourism and travel

Anthea Innes, Nancy McAdam and Joy Watson

Summary

Considering travel and tourism from the perspective of people living with dementia allows us to see what is possible, what should be possible and what adaptations might be required to improve their experience. Research tells us that people living with dementia often face difficulties when going on holiday or travelling, but that the benefits outweigh any challenges. People living with dementia may change how and where they want to go because of difficulties they have either experienced or fear due to their now having dementia. Research also shows that it is possible for tourism providers to make adjustments so that services are accessible. Looking at travel and tourism through the lens of the experiences of people living with dementia allows us to see that it is possible to continue to travel and to enjoy tourism when one has dementia. Tourism and travel providers can enhance the experiences of people living with dementia travelling for leisure purposes by: learning more about dementia; creating an experience that addresses physical and emotional needs; providing help with way-finding. People living with dementia can learn from others with dementia and continue to fulfil their travel and tourism wishes. The challenge for everyone is making dementia-friendly travel and tourism a reality for all.

About the authors and our aims for the chapter

Three people have written this chapter: a professor (Anthea) and two individuals living with dementia. Nancy lives in the Black Isle, a rural area of Scotland, and Joy lives in a suburb of a large English city. We have known each other for some time, meeting at events and conferences in different European countries, and working together in many ways, including presenting together and taking part in community engagement and awareness ventures. We have a common commitment to raising awareness of dementia and helping to shape and inform knowledge to improve the lives of those who may be diagnosed with dementia in the future.

In this chapter we consider travel and tourism through a social inclusion and social citizenship lens (Innes et al. 2004; Bartlett 2021). These are key concepts that promote understanding of living with dementia beyond a focus on the individual's experience of a health condition, taking into account instead the wider social context of living with dementia and how society can respond so as to enable individuals living with dementia to fully participate in social life. Looking at tourism and travel in this way allows us to see what is possible, what should be possible and what adaptations might be required to improve the experiences of people living with dementia.

People often share difficulties they have faced when going on holiday or travelling when they are living with dementia. These difficulties could be compounded by other health conditions or comorbidities, or having healthcare needs arising from other issues – for example, sight, hearing, heart or mobility challenges issues might be more challenging for travel than having dementia. Dementia or other health conditions can influence medical teams to advise against travel creating a tension for the person wishing to travel and medical advice. However, providing certain measures are taken – such as obtaining appropriate quantities of medications necessary for the trip, letters from health providers explaining any medications/conditions and travel insurance – travel can still be possible. Travel and tourism can straddle 'serious leisure' (perhaps a trip to hone one's skills, for example in playing golf) and 'communicative leisure', which may be part of everyday life experiences enabling us to sustain a sense of self and well-being. 'Tourism' refers to trips where an overnight stay is required. So tourism normally involves travelling, perhaps by car, train, boat or aeroplane, to destinations in the country where a person lives or to another country. Research has shown that it is possible for tourism providers to make adjustments so that their services are accessible to those living with dementia and their friends and family who may travel with them (Connell and Page 2020). It also shows that people living with dementia may change their preferred travel options and tourism destinations due to difficulties they have either experienced in the past or fear they might experience in future due to their now having dementia (Innes et al. 2016).

This chapter shares the specific challenges Joy and Nancy have faced when continuing to travel for tourism and leisure. It provides examples of what has made their experiences of travel and tourism worthwhile and of why continuing to travel for holidays and to meet others is important to their sense of well-being. It is also important to their 'social health' (Vernooij-Dassen and Jeon 2016), a term that refers to the idea that participation in the social world can enhance individual well-being. For travel and tourism this relates to how participating in such activities promotes social health through creating a sense of purpose, belonging, adventure and enjoyment. The Covid-19 pandemic led to restrictions on everyone's opportunities for travel, and particularly impacted people living with dementia as travel can be life-enhancing. It is evident from Nancy and Joy's reflections that it will take a great deal of effort and resilience for people living with dementia to feel confident about returning to travelling.

We first provide an overview of what is known from the research relating to travel, tourism and leisure for people living with dementia. We then go on to discuss five issues that draw on the research and on the experiences Nancy and Joy wish to share: the importance of travel and tourism for Nancy and Joy; the importance of travel and tourism for well-being; challenges of travelling alone when living with dementia; supporting independent travel and tourism; reflections and learning from Covid-19 lockdown experiences.

We will end with learning points for those providing tourism travel services, researchers and for people living with dementia and their care partners who wish to continue to pursue tourism and leisure opportunities.

What does the research tell us?

Too often people report difficulties they have faced when going on holiday or travelling for other purposes when they have dementia (Innes et al. 2016; Timmermans et al. 2020). Yet leisure activities away from home have self-reported benefits for the well-being of people living with dementia and their care partners (Fortune et al. 2021). Day trips and holidays are also valued by both the person living with dementia and their care partners (Innes et al. 2016).

Internationally, there has been an increase in research interest in travel and tourism for people living with dementia. We know that more research is required (Klímová 2018) about how to attain 'dementia-friendly tourism' (Page et al. 2015); but what there is already shows us that people living with dementia may change their preferred travel options and tourism destinations due to difficulties they have either experienced or fear due to their now having dementia (Innes et al. 2016). This reflects the awareness we have of vulnerabilities people living with dementia report when outside and away from their homes (Bartlett and Brannelly 2019). Leisure opportunities are key to preserving and making friendships that promote connectedness (Fortune et al. 2021) and therefore the well-being of people living with dementia.

We know travel can become problematic for people living with dementia when they are no longer assessed as being able to drive and when public transport becomes the main way to travel (Scottish Dementia Working Group 2016). It is important to remember to check the requirements where you live in terms of reporting that you have dementia, and to be assessed on a regular basis as safe to continue to drive. When driving is no longer possible, ensuring that any concessionary transport options are explored is important. For example, free or reduced fares can be accessed via disability assessments and other benefits that a person living with dementia may be assessed as being entitled to in their country of residence. Free or reduced cost public travel can help retain the ability to explore new places. A review (Risser et al. 2015) of the experiences of people living with dementia using different forms of public transport concluded that much needs to be done to raise awareness throughout the travel industry about dementia and how to best provide appropriate support. The Scottish Dementia Working Group have created a useful guide (2016) for travelling safely with dementia, produced by people living with dementia to help people living with dementia learn from each other's experiences. However, systemic challenges will remain until businesses address the difficulties their services, or lack thereof, present for those travelling who have a dementia diagnosis.

We know also that people living with dementia wish to participate in leisure activities and dementia-friendly holidays, and that businesses are interested in making their service more dementia-friendly, but that both groups need more support to make this a reality (Timmermans et al. 2020). Care partners and people living with dementia feel that public attitudes towards dementia (Innes et al. 2016; Timmermans et al. 2020) are a barrier to their enjoyment of leisure and holiday activities. Promoting broad knowledge and awareness about dementia, including to tourism, leisure and travel providers, remains vital if the wider agenda of the inclusion of people living with dementia in all aspects of social life is to become a reality. It is important to also consider travel insurance when planning a holiday following a diagnosis of dementia. Some companies may not offer coverage, or be too expensive. But many companies will provide travel insurance. The diagnosis should be disclosed and any worsening of symptoms may need reporting over time. Typical key questions that insurers may ask about dementia are 'Are you travelling with someone or alone?' and 'Are you going to participate in any risky activities when on your trip?' Responses to these questions can influence both whether insurance will be issued and the price quoted. However, it is possible to get travel insurance with age, rather than the dementia diagnosis, often being a factor that might increase the cost of insurance.

How to support tourism providers to improve their offer to people living with dementia?

To make their services user-friendly for those living with dementia and friends and family travelling with them, tourism providers can learn more about dementia (Page et al. 2015; Innes et al. 2016). Guides exist (e.g. VisitEngland 2019) to help businesses with this. Where staff seek to engage and include those with dementia at tourist attractions, such as heritage sites, this can result in experiences which have a positive impact on the self-reported well-being of those with dementia, helping also to strengthen relationships with care partners and supporters through shared enjoyment (Innes et al. 2021). Businesses need to optimize resources available, such as staff and the physical environment, to promote accessibility for people living with dementia and their care partners. However, they face challenges in ensuring that they meet the expectations and needs of people living with dementia, while raising awareness among employees of what is often an invisible condition, to improve customer care (Connell and Page 2020).

Creating a dementia-inclusive society

Helping businesses address the challenges of providing services to people living with dementia is part of a UK (Department of Health 2015) and wider international effort to achieve dementia-friendly, or inclusive, communities (Alzheimer's Disease International 2017). Dementia-inclusive societies are premised on the basis that people living with dementia are offered the same opportunities as everyone else to participate in social life. Travel and tourism are activities enjoyed by many; looking forward to holidays to visit new places, participating in new or age-old favourite activities and visiting friends and family all bring benefits to well-being and social health. Ensuring that people living with dementia can participate in this domain of everyday life, and are supported if required, is part of creating a more inclusive society. People with a diagnosis of dementia do not need to accept that their diagnosis means a lack of independence and rights (Wiersma et al. 2016). Policy directives acknowledge that people living with dementia can actively contribute to and engage in their communities – for example, the Prime Minister's Dementia Challenge in the UK (Department of Health 2015). The ability to travel, visit new places, experience new things or return to favourite haunts falls into the realm of travel, tourism and leisure and is part of everyday life; ensuring that these sectors continue to be available to those living with dementia is therefore clearly important.

The importance of travel and tourism for Joy and Nancy

Research shows that travel, leisure and tourism are important to people living with dementia, offering the opportunity to remain connected, experience new things, go to new places and to have fun (Innes et al. 2016; Timmermans et al. 2020). This is evident too in the views of Nancy and Joy, who enjoy travelling for holidays and also to meet and share their experiences of dementia with other people living with the condition. In their words:

Joy: I really enjoy being out there, I've always been a hands-on person. So, when dementia arrived, I decided to embrace the challenges. I believe it's important to stay connected; tourism is one way of doing that. Travel and freedom are important for my well-being. Having dementia makes travel difficult, but not impossible.

Nancy: Walking scenic walks is something I really enjoy. But I also like sightseeing in new cities, and eating out is an experience I love. A swim in the sea is nice, and also in a pool. Fish and chips are always a favourite for me when I am out and about. And of course, being in company with others is a delight! Travelling, holidays with my family, and meeting others living with dementia at conferences and events in Europe and in Scotland are really important to me. I like to be out and about.

These accounts, from two women living in different contexts, demonstrate that travel and tourism matter to them, in the same way that they do for many, regardless of whether we are living with dementia or not. The outings may be to new places to explore, or familiar walks which bring comfort from their familiarity, but where, for example, the different seasons bring a different view of leaves unfurling in the spring, or the colours of autumn foliage. The important thing is retaining the ability to get outside to familiar and new places giving the opportunity to talk, either by reminiscing or creating new memories.

The importance of travel and tourism for well-being

Maintaining the social health and well-being of people living with dementia is a key concern for policy and practice (Department of Health 2015). Attending different social groups, such as those held at heritage sites, can help achieve well-being (Innes et al. 2021). Well-being can also be achieved through connection with other people, enjoyment of a place (new or familiar) and participation in activities that are fun or fulfilling for the individual, as Nancy and Joy discuss below.

Nancy: My last real memory of travelling to Europe was to Copenhagen, to an Alzheimer Europe conference. My expenses were covered by the Life Changes Trust.[1] I had facial cellulitis at the time and my face was a mess, but it was ok to attend. It was important for me to still be able to participate and meet my friends with dementia from across Europe.

In the past I travelled to France for holidays with friends every year. This year, I visited Rothesay, on the Isle of Bute for a walking holiday with my family. My family picked me up in the car from the Black Isle, we travelled down to Glasgow then got the ferry across. Holidays – with friends and family – are so important to me. The benefits to me are huge, the companionship with people you know well and that know you well. There are so many benefits to travelling – I enjoy being outside, out in the fresh air. But my travel for dementia advocacy purposes, various conferences in Europe over the years and in Scotland, is really important. I like planning events with other people living with dementia, sharing experiences with others in similar circumstances from different places. Seeing people face to face is very important. I remember a trip to Ireland and talking about experiences of living with dementia in rural areas. The event grabbed the media attention and I was asked to talk to the press. What was so good was that evening sitting down with the other speakers in the local pub for a meal, and we appeared on the evening news! We were sitting eating and our faces came up on the big TV. The bar tender turned it up so we could all hear. Dementia holidays were an annual event I looked forward to until Covid-19 enforced lockdowns. Other people living with dementia sometimes point out things, and others with dementia can be very perceptive of other people's needs. One activity that sticks in my mind was white-water rafting – that was a

Joy: real adventure. It was very exciting being in the water in the Findhorn – getting soaked – it was quite exhilarating!

Joy: The most exciting holidays I've had have been with a dementia holiday company. The emphasis is on adventure. Now me being an adrenalin junkie means I can continue to enjoy doing crazy things like swimming in a freezing cold lake in just my underwear. Health and safety meant someone had to swim with me and a member of staff got the short straw. These holidays are so dementia-friendly it's amazing, from pouring your tea at breakfast to stop me scalding myself, to reminding me to take my walking stick on our daily adventures. Another massive bonus is that I'm picked up from my front door and returned to my home once the holiday has finished.

Riding the white-knuckle rides at the theme parks is my idea of heaven. The zip wire in Wales has got to be one of the most exhilarating experiences I've had. Yes, I enjoy walking, visiting garden centres and national parks, but put me on a speedboat in Southport and I am one happy bunny. I don't do sitting on a beach or soaking up the sun by the pool, my idea of relaxing is jet skiing from a beach in Spain.

When people living with dementia continue to travel for leisure and tourism, it can enable inclusion, maintain skills and means there is a continued opportunity to do enjoyable things.

Maintaining skills and doing what you enjoy

Research – and common sense – tells us how important it is to be able to maintain skills and participate in activities that are enjoyable (Innes et al. 2016; Wiersma et al. 2016). Different kinds of leisure – both serious and communicative – may intersect when people living with dementia travel, as Joy demonstrates through sharing her memories below.

Joy: Before my dementia deteriorated, I enjoyed camping. I would drive myself to the campsite, having informed the owners of my disability, a must if you are staying alone.

I must admit, I do tend to stick to organized trips these days, and a Scottish tour company has proven to be exceptional. It's a coach company that caters for my needs, picking me up from my local bus station, allocating me a seat for the duration of the trip, organizing excursions every day and evening entertainment. What more could you want? Unlike the adventure holidays, these getaways are more sedate.

I think the best support you can have are people who know a little about the condition. People who are willing to let you try out-of-the-box things. People who encourage you to live well despite the dementia. The holiday company [providing specialized holiday provision in the UK for people living with dementia] team could have said 'No, you can't swim in the lake', but instead they supported me to do it. Sometimes it's about taking calculated risks. I don't remember very much of any of my trips due to the effects of the dementia, but I will always remember that swim and the feeling it gave me.

The right to take risks to promote enjoyment and well-being is one that can be contentious; professionals may seek to avoid risk and employ risk-aversion strategies. However, as Joy's experiences and government guidance demonstrates, the right to make a choice and to take risks is important when one has dementia (Department of Health 2010), even though it can be difficult to find the balance between protecting against perceived harm while respecting individual personal rights, choices and freedom. Indeed, if medical advice is not to travel it can be important to consider if this is due to a fear of risk, and therefore what can be done to mitigate perceived risks – e.g. obtaining the correct travel insurance or finding a support person to travel with.

Challenges of travelling alone when living with dementia

There may be an assumption that a dementia diagnosis can make travelling alone so difficult that a travel companion is required. This may in fact be the case in some instances, for some people or for some trips. However, Nancy and Joy have both continued to travel alone and overcome the challenges they experienced.

Joy: Planning one's journey and venue is imperative to avoid potential problems. I have encountered some difficulties while travelling. On a train journey from London to Manchester, I was surrounded by a group of unruly youngsters. I couldn't get help as I was hemmed in. I phoned my carer who then contacted the train manager. Sadly, the frightening situation was not resolved and I stayed like that until I got to my station. However, I wasn't put off by this experience; the enjoyment of tourism and travel always outweighs the occasional hiccup.

Getting lost in hotels is par for the course for me too. I've lost count of how many times I've left my keys on the dining table. The panic that envelopes me at these times is dispersed if the staff are understanding. I try desperately to remember my room number and feel somewhat embarrassed when I can't.

Nancy: One of the most frustrating experiences I had was at an airport. I had requested assistance and they decided that meant me sitting in a wheelchair and getting wheeled to the gate. Even though I can walk! I wanted to go to a shop to buy a present, Scottish whisky, to take with me to give to my friend I was visiting, but I couldn't do this as

I had been asked to stay in a wheelchair while at the airport and I couldn't find the shop on my own. Putting me in a wheelchair even when I am physically mobile, and I couldn't go anywhere as I was told not to move. This experience made me more disabled than I actually am! Assistance should be tailored to individual needs. But a 'catch-all' approach of putting those who request assistance in a wheelchair was the practice I experienced, and it was not a good experience! I find airports more difficult generally; train stations tend to be easier to navigate – they are well signposted and, of course, I have used trains regularly throughout my life and so they are still familiar to me.

Supporting independent travel and tourism

As discussed above, finding ways for travel providers to enable independent travel has been acknowledged as important. But as Nancy and Joy share, one of the best ways to overcome difficulties may be for others involved in a journey to assist.

Nancy: One of the best things to help with travelling is when other people think about and anticipate what people living with dementia might need. An experience I had with a DEEP[2] event I was invited to was very good. The idea was that a group of women were given the chance to speak together about what they are concerned about, in a setting that was comfortable for speaking and sharing experiences. It is so important to have the opportunity to share with people who are friendly and welcoming and helpful to everyone.

In this instance, the travel arrangements were all made and communicated clearly to me to help make the experience stress free. It really feels so much better when someone sends the details of timings of the journey, and the bus numbers, and the places where to change; it takes some of the stress out of it when travelling alone. Where I live is rural; I need to get either the community car or a taxi to the airport. Inverness airport is easy as it is small, but landing somewhere else, like London, that can be difficult. But knowing where to go and knowing someone is waiting to pick you up, that they will come and find you if you don't appear when you should after the plane has landed – that really gives me peace of mind!

I also sometimes stay in Birmingham with a dementia holiday provider, and it is really user-friendly. They have thought about what might go wrong, so that when you come to stay the problems are already resolved. Simple things like signposting to help you find your way around is really important. Staying in a hotel room can be difficult – for example, how to work a shower in a different environment. I stayed in one place where I couldn't control the temperature in the shower and scalded my skin. Luckily I was sharing a room with another person with dementia and she was very good and managed to help me work out how to use the shower. Having someone there to help can be very reassuring.

The other thing that really helps me travel is my local community car scheme. When they give you a lift they wait outside until they know the meeting is taking place.

Being able to drive on my own land down to the main road and the bus stop is really important to me, even though I am not allowed to drive on public roads because of my dementia. I have a friend's old four-wheel drive now; it's an automatic gearbox and so really easy to drive, and goes over all the bumps of my track easily. I love it!

Joy: The majority of my trips have been very positive. I've acquired a disability lanyard which has proved very helpful when travelling from my local airport. Most airport staff are familiar with the bright sunflower lanyard and are available to help when I need help. I wouldn't be able to travel and stay in hotel accommodation without a support worker. My support worker is invaluable; she encourages me to remain independent without smothering me.

I love driving, and with the help of my sat nav I can negotiate most journeys. The only problems I encounter is when there is a diversion and the sat nav is slow to inform me of the changes. My car breakdown membership gives me the confidence to venture out. I have always been independent and I want to be independent for as long as I can.

Joy and Nancy's accounts show that, although travelling independently can be difficult, the difficulties can be overcome with forward planning, enjoying the experience and/or receiving assistance from others, and a good degree of personal perseverance.

Reflections and learning from Covid-19 lockdown experiences

Reflecting on their experiences of constraints to their freedom of movement and the ability to travel demonstrates the impact Covid-19 has had for Joy and Nancy, something that has also been written about by others living with dementia (e.g. Rochford-Brennan and Keogh 2020).

Nancy: Covid-19 has restricted travel and it is terrible that Covid-19 has stopped everything, as it is now difficult to even remember some of the things that have been lost. It feels like a backward step. I have still been going to a mindfulness group locally and that really helps. I think that it is crucial to continue to get out and see things to keep awareness and use existing skills. Since lockdown – and 18 months is a long time! – I have changed what I do. I've had to read for entertainment and go out walking locally with family when they visited. We have been to different places. We used walk maps and tried new local walks. This was really important, to just get out, and be with others, to be doing something different.

I am feeling a bit tentative about travelling again. Even just yesterday, I had a difficult experience. I wanted to join my local walking group again, and got the community car to pick me up and take me to the usual meeting place. But they had changed the meeting place since the last time I went, and so I ended up at the wrong place and missed the walk. I've already missed a lot during Covid-19 restriction times, and this was really disappointing. I felt quite sad and stupid for being at the wrong place!

I have concerns about travelling again as it may be more and more difficult as I am out of practice. I think I will need to relearn how to travel again and use the skills I had before. I have not travelled alone for 18 months now, and so travelling alone again is a bit frightening. I keep thinking, can I still do it? Can I remember what to do?

Joy: Where I live, during lockdown we could access outside spaces on video – we had a six-week programme visiting farms and felt like we were getting to know the animals. And although this was second best, it was educational and it was the next best thing and helped. Walking groups, every other week we went on a walk on video, but we were introduced to the trees and the plants and it felt like we were travelling outside. It was a compromise and a compromise worth doing. Because we could look at the outdoors it gave us hope! Some of the animals we named and got to know on the videos we have now been able to meet in reality, and go to the places we visited on the video. Doing that gave us normality again! We could interact, stroke and talk to the animals, and so it was an uplifting experience and I felt normal again.

The experiences of Joy and Nancy demonstrate challenges arising from Covid-19 measures. However, these are challenges they are prepared to tackle, as the benefits to their well-being of getting out, meeting others and doing things they enjoy trumps any apprehension they feel about having to relearn rusty or forgotten skills.

Opening up possibilities

Considering travel and tourism through a social inclusion and social citizenship lens allows us to see what is possible, what should be possible and what adaptations might be required to improve the experiences of people living with dementia when they travel. Nancy and Joy's personal accounts above illustrate what is possible to achieve, while acknowledging the difficulties faced.

It is possible to continue to travel and to enjoy tourism when one has dementia. Nancy and Joy have both travelled widely to share their experiences of dementia at conferences in the UK and beyond. They have also continued to enjoy holidays with friends and family, as well as those designed for people with dementia. Both travel purposes, for leisure and to meet others with dementia, are very important; remaining connected with family and friends and making and maintaining new friendships with others with a dementia diagnosis are very empowering. Equally travelling can be a way for the person living with dementia to connect with their spouse, family and friends and to make and share memories together. Importantly, travel can be enjoyable for the person providing support as well as for the person living with dementia.

Tourism and travel providers can enhance experiences of travel. As has been noted above, information is available for heritage settings (e.g. Visit England 2019) and transport providers (Scottish Dementia Working Group 2016) to help guide their practices so that they offer an accessible and enriching experience for those with dementia who might travel with them or visit tourist attractions or destinations. The challenge remains to make dementia-friendly travel and tourism a reality for all. The learning points below have been developed together by the co-authors of this chapter. Implementing them in practice would give any service or business wishing to meet this challenge a great start.

So what does this mean in practice?

For those supporting or enabling the involvement in leisure of people living with dementia

* *Learn as much as you can about dementia.* As a start, make sure all staff participate in a dementia-awareness course. This can be developed to include thinking about having a linked named person with a higher level of knowledge to provide extra support and information to clients living with dementia seeking to arrange travel and to colleagues with more basic levels of awareness. The Flight Centre is one company that has provided dedicated support to people living with dementia and which has previously partnered with the Alzheimer Society in the UK and encouraged its staff to become dementia friends to ensure they were dementia aware and inclusive and responsive to the needs of people living with dementia seeking advice on travel bookings. Meeting the needs of people affected by dementia, be it the person living with the condition or the care partner, isn't rocket science. The desire to help someone to have a good experience should be paramount. Bear in mind, this may be the last trip they are able to go on. Empathy is key to relating to others and communicating well. Remember that people with dementia may forget the facts. They may forget what part of the country they visited, they may not remember the details of the venue, but chances are they will remember how sitting on the sea wall with an ice cream made them feel. The part of the brain that retains feelings and emotions functions better and longer than the factual part of the brain.

- *Create an experience that addresses physical and emotional needs.* If operators are committed to giving a positive experience to people living with dementia when travelling, if they provide more than a comfy bed and good food, if they offer menus that are understandable – perhaps by using larger font and images – if they have thought about providing instructions in a hotel room to operate the shower or the lamps: if they do these things, more people living with dementia are likely to travel again.
- *Provide help with wayfinding.* Look at the signposting in hotels or other public venues like airports and railway stations. If good systems are in place, for example signs that include words and images and that are placed at eye-level and in positions that catch the eye, that means everything happens easily, and saves the person with dementia (and anyone else!) having to think about it.

For people living with dementia

Based on their experiences of travelling for tourism and leisure and for advocacy, Joy and Nancy share their learning points for others living with dementia about travel and tourism.

Joy: I'd say to anyone with a disability, put in place the support you need and go for it. Making memories is so important. Try to get some form of record of where you've been and what you've done: photos or videos are great – they may help jog your memory later in your dementia journey.

Nancy: What you don't know you don't know, so you have to ask others to find out. Don't be scared to speak up – ask for help. Don't hesitate, ask for help as soon as you need it! Ask for directions, look for visual clues to help you find your way around and work out what's happening. Still travel, don't be put off, don't let the disability stop you.

For researchers

- Be sure to include the views and perspectives of people living with dementia.

Endnotes

1 In 2022, Age Scotland and About Dementia became National Legacy Partners for the Life Changes Trust. For more information about the work of the Trust, and to access legacy resources, visit https://www.ageuk.org.uk/scotland/what-we-do/dementia/about-dementia/resources/

2 DEEP (Dementia Engagement and Empowerment Project) is a UK network of organizations for people living with dementia. For more information on the DEEP organization, please see: www.dementiavoices.org.uk/

References

Alzheimer's Disease International (2017) *Dementia Friendly Communities Global Developments*. London: Alzheimer's Disease International. Available at: https://www.alzint.org/u/dfc-developments.pdf (accessed 17 August 2021).

Bartlett, R. (2021) Inclusive (social) citizenship and persons with dementia, *Disability & Society*, 37(7): 1129–45.

Bartlett, R. and Brannelly, T. (2019) On being outdoors: How people with dementia experience and deal with vulnerabilities, *Social Science and Medicine*, 235(5): 112236.

Connell, J. and Page, S. (2020) Tourism, ageing and the demographic time bomb – the implications of dementia for the visitor economy: A perspective paper, *Tourism Review*, 75(1): 81–5.

Department of Health (2010) *'Nothing Ventured, Nothing Gained': Risk Guidance for Dementia*. London: DoH. Available at: https://assets.publishing.service.gov.uk/government/uploads/system/uploads/attachment_data/file/215960/dh_121493.pdf (accessed 12 October 2021).

Department of Health (2015) *Prime Minister's Challenge on Dementia 2020*. London: DoH. Available at: https://assets.publishing.service.gov.uk/government/uploads/system/uploads/attachment_data/file/414344/pm-dementia2020.pdf (accessed 3 August 2021).

Fortune, D., Whyte, C. and Genoe, R. (2021) The interplay between leisure, friendship, and dementia, *Dementia*, 20(6): 2041–56.

Innes, A., Archibald, C. and Murphy, C. (eds) (2004) *Dementia: An Inclusive Future?: Marginalised Groups and Marginalised Areas of Dementia Research, Care and Practice*. London: Jessica Kingsley Publishers.

Innes, A., Page, S.J. and Cutler, C. (2016) Barriers to leisure participation for people with dementia and their carers: An exploratory analysis of carer and people with dementia's experiences, *Dementia*, 15(6): 1643–65.

Innes, A., Scholar, H.F., Haragalova, J. and Sharma, M. (2021) 'You come because it is an interesting place': The impact of attending a heritage programme on the well-being of people living with dementia and their care partners, *Dementia*, 20(6): 2133–51.

Klímová, B. (2018) Tourists with dementia – a unique challenge for the tourism industry, *Social Sciences and Humanities*, 26(1): 583–8.

Page, S.J., Innes, A. and Cutler, C. (2015) Developing dementia-friendly tourism destinations: An exploratory analysis, *Journal of Travel Research*, 54(4): 467–81.

Risser, R., Lexell, E.M., Bell, D. et al. (2015) Use of local public transport among people with cognitive impairments – a literature review, *Transportation Research, Part F*, 29: 83–97.

Rochford-Brennan, H. and Keogh, F. (2020) Giving voice to those directly affected by the COVID-19 pandemic – the experience and reflections of a person with dementia, *HRB Open Research*, 3. Available at: https://doi.org/10.12688/hrbopenres.13063.1 (accessed 10 January 2023).

Scottish Dementia Working Group (2016) *Travelling Safely with Dementia*. Available at: https://www.alzscot.org/sites/default/files/2019-07/Travelling-with-dementia-V4-07.09.16.pdf (accessed 17 August 2021).

Timmermans, O., van de Velde, I. and Matthijsse, M. (2020) Perception of people living with dementia and entrepreneurs on dementia-friendly leisure activities in society, *Journal of Sociology*, 4(4): 130–49.

Vernooij-Dassen, M. and Jeon, Y. (2016) Social health and dementia: The power of human capabilities, *International Psychogeriatrics*, 28(5): 701–3.

VisitEngland (2019) *Dementia-Friendly Tourism: A Practical Guide for Businesses.* London: VisitEngland. Available at: https://www.visitbritain.org/sites/default/ files/vb-corporate/business-hub/resources/dementia_friendly_guide_for_tourism_ businesses.pdf (accessed 16 August 2021).

Wiersma, E.C., O'Connor, D., Loiselle, L. et al. (2016) Creating space for citizenship: The impact of group structure on validating the voices of people with dementia, *Dementia*, 15(3): 414–33.

9 Resisting stigma

Rebecca Genoe and Darla Fortune

Summary

We explore stigma, or negative opinions and beliefs people have about dementia. These include incorrect information that suggests people living with dementia cannot make choices, finish simple tasks, and are no longer interested in daily activities, such as leisure. Because of these incorrect beliefs, people living with dementia may feel lonely, isolated and like they do not belong. They may begin to believe these negative beliefs are true and stop doing their favourite leisure activities, and/or stop spending time with family and friends and doing things that bring them joy. When this happens, people living with dementia may feel even more isolated. But research suggests that engaging in leisure helps change people's negative beliefs about dementia into more positive beliefs. Therefore, we look at ways leisure can help people living with dementia experience dignity and feel appreciated. For example, people have many abilities and often wish to contribute to their communities. If leisure is meaningful and offers them a chance to use their strengths, people living with dementia may make new friends or maintain previous friendships. They may be able to change negative opinions about dementia by showing others they have strengths and abilities, thoughts and feelings that should be considered. This chapter offers recommendations for ensuring people living with dementia have access to personally meaningful leisure experiences. For example:

- having opportunities to communicate their leisure interests to friends, family and leisure providers, and discuss together what resources and support would help them maintain meaningful leisure experiences
- for friends and care partners to seek ways to support them to continue to engage in the leisure experiences they most enjoy
- for leisure providers to recognize that quality leisure experiences can go a long way to resisting stigma and supporting people with dementia to sustain their place in everyday life.

Introduction

Leisure is 'a space where there is room for the self to expand beyond what it is told it should be' (Wearing 1998:146)

Negative attitudes and assumptions about dementia may limit opportunities for leisure. However, meaningful and supported leisure experiences help people living with dementia resist these perspectives and alter such negative beliefs on both personal and societal levels. Wearing's quote, above, celebrates the freedom inherent in leisure to be who we want to be, rather than what we are told we should be. In contrast, discourse on dementia tends to focus on loss and decline. It tells us that someone living with dementia is no longer there, is no longer capable and can no longer experience meaning in life (Mitchell et al. 2013). Yet people living with dementia do experience life after diagnosis (Genoe 2009). They continue to pursue meaningful leisure, they uphold and celebrate relationships with others and they make a difference as socially active citizens in their communities (Genoe 2009; Fortune et al. 2021). As such, they directly contravene negative attitudes about dementia.

This chapter reports on research, situated in Canada, that we undertook to explore the role of leisure for people who are living with dementia, including how they may use leisure to resist stigma. In the chapter, we explore dementia-related stigma and its impacts on individuals living with dementia. Next, we consider whether stigma can be resisted during time spent engaging in leisure. Then we provide examples highlighting leisure opportunities that have enabled resistance among people living with dementia.

Dementia-related stigma

Erving Goffman articulated the concept of stigma in the 1960s. Stigma occurs when people are devalued based on particular characteristics which, in turn, prevent their full participation in society (Goffman 1968). Dementia-related stigma occurs when people living with dementia are devalued due to their diagnosis, and are no longer included in all aspects of their communities, families or groups of friends. Research conducted by the Alzheimer Society of Canada (2017) highlights the impact of dementia-related stigma. In their study, 61 per cent of people living with dementia reported being ignored or dismissed by others; 60 per cent reported not having access to appropriate supports or services; and 59 per cent reported being taken advantage of. The same study also noted that 54 per cent of Canadians believe they would be avoided or rejected due to a dementia diagnosis.

Western society values younger people over older people, equates youth with ability, attractiveness and intelligence, and assumes older adults are frail and incompetent. These ageist assumptions perpetuate dementia-related stigma by associating dementia with loss and decline, rather than experiences of meaning and joy (Mitchell et al. 2013). The implicit message in these assumptions is that a person living with dementia can no longer make decisions, is no longer capable and, in many cases, is no longer considered a person. These assumptions are upheld when terms such as 'the living dead' or 'zombies' (Mitchell et al. 2013) are used to describe people living with dementia. Swaffer

(2014) described her experience of attending an international dementia conference where language such as 'demented', 'sufferers', 'subjects', 'victims' and 'not all there' (p. 711) was used to describe people living with dementia, perpetuating negative connotations about what it is like to live with the diagnosis.

Negative attitudes and assumptions about dementia can have a significant impact on the lives of people living with it. They can lead to negative feelings such as shame, guilt and even abandonment (Swaffer 2014). A person living with dementia may begin to believe these negative assumptions, internalize them, and then may choose to reduce their social contacts (Swaffer 2014). Indeed, a UK survey of older adults living with dementia found that 33 per cent of respondents had lost friends because of their diagnosis, reducing levels of informal social support (Kane and Cook 2013). Additionally, stigma can lead to lack of access to support from a person's community and healthcare system (Benbow and Jolley 2012). For example, people living with dementia may be labelled or described in stigmatizing ways based on behaviours or needs. Consequently, healthcare professionals may not take the health concerns of individuals seriously. Stigma may influence decisions about disclosing one's diagnosis, as this can lead to disregard for personal feelings, preferences and abilities, along with loss of opportunity to engage with one's community – compromising the social citizenship of the person concerned (O'Connor et al. 2018).

Impact of stigma on leisure

Other chapters in this book highlight the valuable role leisure plays in the lives of people living with dementia. However, dementia-related stigma may reduce opportunities for leisure. In fact, results from the UK survey mentioned previously showed that 51 per cent of respondents believed that people living with dementia were unable to engage with their communities. Further, 53 per cent believed there was a lack of appropriate community-based leisure opportunities for people living with dementia (Kane and Cook 2013). Since people living with dementia may consider negative beliefs about dementia to be true, and since they often miss out on opportunities to participate in society, they tend to experience a reduction in meaningful leisure engagement. As dementia-related stigma leads to decreases in engagement with friends and family, people living with dementia may withdraw from these relationships and experience isolation (Kane and Cook 2013). This could lead to the loss of social leisure experiences vital for a sense of belonging, enjoyment and social citizenship. People living with dementia may feel they are no longer welcome to participate in previously enjoyed social leisure – for example, Fortune and McKeown (2016) explored the experiences of people taking part in the Memory Boosters Social Club. Study participants felt excluded from their friendship groups following a diagnosis of dementia and were no longer invited to attend group leisure activities (see Vignette 9.1, below: Cecelia's experience of dementia-related stigma).

Vignette 9.1: Cecelia's experience of dementia-related stigma

The following is a fictionalized account of the experience of dementia-related stigma, deriving from the stories of several research participants who shared their experiences of leisure and memory loss (adapted from Genoe 2009).

Cecelia has been living with early-stage dementia for about three years. She left her job when she was diagnosed, but she lives independently in her own apartment with the support of family members. She advocates for people living with dementia and enjoys several leisure activities that help keep her mind and body active. Yet she finds others no longer see her as a capable, independent person. They assume that Cecelia can no longer look after herself. Her family discourages her from taking the bus to the mall by herself even though Cecelia is confident that she can do it on her own. Her family tells her, 'Don't go to the mall by yourself, because you could wander somewhere.' Cecelia feels frustrated that she is missing one of her favourite leisure activities, but her family's assumptions cause her to question her own abilities, even though she still does plenty of leisure activities by herself. Just last week Cecelia went for a walk but the neighbours, aware of her diagnosis, didn't think she should be out alone and called Cecelia's children to tell them she was outside.

Sometimes even Cecelia's close friends don't treat her with the same respect they used to. Her friend Martha doesn't call her much any more. When she does, she talks to Cecelia as if she is a child and tells her what she should and shouldn't do. When they do get together, Martha is overprotective – she does things for Cecelia instead of allowing her to do them herself. All of these instances of stigma shake Cecelia's confidence. She starts to question whether she can go to the mall or for a walk in her neighbourhood by herself and then misses leisure opportunities. She feels frustrated when her family and friends make assumptions about her abilities or do things for her rather than supporting her independence: 'It's very frustrating, even makes me angry. But I don't want to say anything because I know their intent is good.'

In addition to withdrawal from social groups, loss of leisure engagement may occur when leisure service providers fail to put supports into place for people living with dementia to remain engaged in leisure within their communities. People living with dementia may benefit from adaptations to meaningful leisure opportunities, such as incorporating flexibility to account for individual needs and preferences (Motto-Ochoa et al. 2021) and ensuring familiarity with an activity or setting (Fortune et al. 2021). If leisure service providers fail to recognize the need for adaptations, they may perpetuate stigma and exclude people living with dementia from engaging in meaningful leisure. When the strengths, abilities, interests and needs of people living with dementia are not considered, leisure environments and programmes may not be comfortable or welcoming, and this could lead to a reduction in leisure participation. It is therefore important for leisure services, healthcare providers and others who support people living with dementia to reflect on their assumptions about dementia and how they may be supporting or compromising opportunities for social citizenship (see the next section).

Reflective questions for leisure service and healthcare providers working with people living with dementia

For leisure service and/or healthcare providers it is important to explore, recognize and grapple with biases and negative assumptions that may be held regarding dementia. Consider the following questions in checking your own assumptions about dementia.

1 What biases or assumptions do I see that can affect people living with dementia?
2 What assumptions do I hold about dementia? Where do these assumptions come from?
3 How might I be projecting these views within my professional life?
4 How can I support inclusion, belonging and citizenship among people living with dementia?
5 How can I support people living with dementia to resist dementia-related stigma through their engagement in leisure?

(Adapted from Genoe and Whyte 2015)

Leisure as resistance to stigma

While stigma can have a negative impact on the lives of people living with dementia and may even limit opportunities for engaging in meaningful leisure, leisure itself may serve to counteract this stigma. A key characteristic of leisure is that we can make our own choices about when, how and where we spend our leisure time. Our leisure is often separated from tasks we are obligated to perform. The freedom inherent in leisure makes it an ideal space for resisting the power structures and ideologies within society that may serve to disadvantage some groups over others. These ideologies include beliefs about ageing that favour physical attractiveness and associate health with younger people, and beliefs about dementia that focus on decline instead of strengths and well-being.

Resistance can be described as actions that individuals or groups take to increase their freedom of choice and personal control (Shaw 2006). Resistance takes a variety of forms. Acts of resistance may be individual and/or collective. They can also be either intentional or unintentional (see Table 9.1).

Table 9.1 Types of resistance (Shaw 2006)

Type of resistance	Definition
Individual	When one person resists their personal situation
Collective	The act of a group against people or groups who have power to make decisions that impact their lives – when an act of resistance benefits others
Intentional	When individuals or groups choose to resist powerful groups or individuals or society's beliefs by behaving in a particular way
Unintentional	When individuals engage in behaviours that resist ideologies without intending to

For example, suppose Linda, who is living with dementia, has received comments from members of her book club that she cannot keep up with the discussion. Over time Linda notices book club members stop inviting her to meetings because of their negative views of dementia (stigma). Linda may then *resist* these negative attitudes by *intentionally* starting a new, inclusive book club that celebrates abilities and strengths, rather than upholding our society's negative beliefs about dementia and book club members' assumptions that someone living with dementia has nothing to contribute. The new book club members then *collectively* resist negative beliefs about dementia by showing others and themselves that they can engage in lively debate about the agreed upon books. Thus, joining and participating in the book club is more than just an enjoyable leisure activity; it is also an act of resistance against negative perceptions about people living with dementia.

Indeed, leisure is a means of resisting discrimination, such as sexism or ageism, that leads to oppression among particular groups of people (Shaw 2006). For example, engagement in meaningful leisure can be a way for women to resist societal expectations regarding how they should behave (Shaw 2006). Older adults resist ageist stereotypes that value youth over experience by selecting leisure activities that are meaningful, rather than spending time on activities that society deems appropriate for people their age (Genoe and Whyte 2015).

When older adults resist ageist assumptions, they also experience empowerment, self-confidence, pride, self-expression and control over their situations (Wearing 1998). While research exploring leisure as resistance among people living with dementia is limited, evidence suggests that engaging in meaningful leisure may indeed provide space for people living with dementia to resist stigma (see Vignette 9.1). Since leisure is a context where we focus on strengths and abilities rather than losses, for people living with dementia and their supporters leisure may be used to demonstrate to others that society's focus on loss and decline fails to acknowledge that life following diagnosis can be meaningful, joyful and even hopeful.

Vignette 9.1 continued: How Cecelia uses leisure to resist dementia-related stigma

Despite Cecelia's experience of stigma, she wants to change other people's beliefs about dementia. She reminds her family and friends that she still has many capabilities. She tells them, 'I think I would fare better if you treat me like you always did.' Cecelia's advocacy work helps her show others that she still has a lot to give to the world. She says her family and friends believed her diagnosis meant she was already in the final stages of dementia, but she teaches them that their perspective is inaccurate. Further, Cecelia's leisure activities demonstrate to others that she has many strengths and abilities: 'My leisure activities show that I still have a lot to give. If I show my friends my crocheting, it's amazing.' Cecelia feels that she can cope well with dementia, and when she maintains her leisure activities, others start to see that she does so. Cecelia also seeks out new opportunities to learn and build skills through her leisure. She learned how to use a computer after her diagnosis to stay in touch with others and to support her advocacy. She started reading for fun and tried new games, like crokinole (a board game) and bocce ball (a lawn game), after diagnosis.

Cecelia uses her leisure for resistance both intentionally, as she displays her remaining abilities to others, and unintentionally as she embraces new opportunities, particularly when others might assume that she cannot learn or try new things. Cecelia resists negative assumptions about dementia through leisure collectively through her advocacy work. She also unintentionally resists negative assumptions when she simply plays cards or crokinole with a friend for fun, while also demonstrating that she can learn new things. By remaining socially active and connected to others, Celia is also reinforcing her social citizenship.

In the next section, we aim to contribute to a more positive view of dementia by sharing examples from recent research demonstrating how people living with dementia may use leisure as a space to resist dementia-related stigma as a means of upholding their social citizenship.

Examples of leisure as a space to resist dementia-related stigma

There are numerous examples depicting how time spent in leisure can enable resistance to stigma by contributing to valued identities for people living with dementia. For instance, Noone and Jenkins (2018) described how participation in a community garden enabled people living with dementia to work together to achieve shared goals, bond over a mutual interest in gardening and relate to one another as citizens beyond their shared dementia diagnoses. As Noone and Jenkins (2018) explained, when pleasurable leisure experiences focus on mutually enjoyable interests rather than the dementia diagnosis, they afford people living with dementia the opportunity to resist stigma by expressing valued aspects of their identity that had become less prominent after their diagnosis. For example, a participant in their study who was a lifelong gardener gained recognition for his gardening abilities and reclaimed this aspect of his identity.

As another example of ways identity-affirming leisure experiences can help to resist stigma, Sass et al. (2021) described how sport memories groups, consisting of inclusive sports-based reminiscence and physical activities for men living with dementia, highlight the importance of inclusive groups for helping individuals to remain socially active and preserve their identities. By combining social interaction with opportunities to revisit life-defining memories, these groups enabled men to express their masculine identities and supported a sense of belonging and social citizenship by reinforcing a shared identity through familiar experiences (e.g. discussing their football days) with like-minded individuals. Shared activities (e.g. playing bocce ball and darts) also enabled some men to contribute to the group by taking other men in the group under their wings.

Exploring the possibility of golf as a dementia-friendly activity, Norval et al. (2021) demonstrated that when personally meaningful leisure activities are person-centred and incorporate elements of support, people living with dementia continue to derive joy from their participation. Norval et al. (2021) examined a social enterprise called *Golden Golfers*, which aims to make golf more accessible regardless of age or skill, and which has a particular focus on supporting people living with dementia through pairing participants with staff members (golfing buddies) to assist them in playing golf and providing companionship. *Golden Golfers* provides an example of how leisure activities can be modified in ways that challenge the stigma surrounding the types of leisure activities deemed appropriate for people living with dementia. Easy-to-follow instructions, reducing the pace and providing frequent reminders may help modify activities so that they are more inclusive. Focusing on cooperation instead of competition is another useful way to support inclusion. As Norval et al. (2021) argued, when such activities are inclusive and supportive, people living with dementia can continue to experience a pleasurable pastime with its associated physical and social benefits while being free from judgement.

The potential for leisure to bring about enjoyment that upholds identity and dignity is not limited to people living with dementia who remain in the community. Isene et al. (2022) observed hospital patients living with dementia in a psychiatric department for four months. While the patients regularly conveyed feeling insignificant and burdensome, it was also observed that leisure activities such as baking, gardening and reading poetry provided experiences that counteracted negative feelings. By reconnecting patients with their former occupational identities through leisure (e.g. poet, teacher, gardener), and helping nurture social relationships – which are often lost following a diagnosis of dementia – these activities contributed to patients' experiences of dignity and significance. Additionally, when patients participated in familiar lifelong traditions such as singing Christmas carols and baking Christmas cookies, the study's authors observed experiences of belonging.

Examples provided thus far show a range of leisure experiences that help resist dementia-related stigma by supporting people living with dementia to continue to participate in meaningful experiences that enhance identity, support freedom and enjoyment and help maintain social citizenship. However, we cannot overlook the significant roles that family, friends and other individuals play when it comes to people living with dementia being able to maintain meaningful experiences. As Fortune et al. (2021) found, friends are instrumental to individuals living with dementia maintaining their leisure engagement. They also found that leisure experiences in turn support the maintenance of friendships for individuals with dementia. Maintaining friendships helps people retain a sense of meaning. Individuals living with dementia who receive support and encouragement from their friendships are able to experience meaning and sustain valued aspects of their identities. This is not a one-way exchange; friends of people living with dementia also derive meaning from mutually enjoyable experiences (Fortune et al. 2021).

A participant in the study by Fortune et al. (2021) – research where individuals with dementia and their friends and family discussed potential interplays between leisure, friendship and dementia – spoke appreciatively about visiting her friend living with dementia in a long-term care home. She described these visits as enjoyable because she was able to spend quality time with her friend while engaging in leisure programming happening within the home. Particularly noteworthy visits involved live music that both friends delighted in, and quiet time spent together sharing a chocolate bar. Additionally, since both friends shared a love of dogs, meaningful visits would also involve time spent at a nearby dog park. As this example suggests, participants in this study highlighted ways mutual leisure interests were at the root of their friendships and noted how they were able to preserve their friendships by continuing to do things both enjoyed. The continuation of friendships and mutually enjoyable leisure experiences help ward off stigma by supporting people living with dementia to maintain meaning in their lives.

In addition to friendships, social interactions with other people living with dementia also contribute to meaningful experiences that help people derive joy without fear of judgement or stigma. Fortune and McKeown (2016), for example, conducted research on a peer-led social group for individuals living with dementia and their care partners and discovered that the creation of an accepting and nonjudgemental environment enabled members to experience meaningful social interactions while avoiding stigma. The social group created this environment by not pointing out when someone said or did something out of place and by being patient when individuals used repetitive speech. As Fortune and McKeown (2016) discovered, when leisure spaces bring individuals who have traditionally been stigmatized and excluded into community life, there are greater opportunities for people to establish social connections with others that can result in experiences of inclusion, belonging and social citizenship.

Motta-Ochoa et al.'s (2021) study also highlighted ways community organizations supporting people living with dementia can create inclusive environments conducive to experiences of belonging and social citizenship. They explored how staff working within an activity centre attended by individuals with dementia supported everyone to feel included. Findings from this study captured ways staff normalized dementia-related behaviours (e.g. repetitive speech and restlessness) by accepting these symptoms as 'part of life' and modelling inclusion and compassion. This modelling approach led some individuals with dementia to take on caregiving roles by supporting someone who experienced more symptoms than they did. The authors also observed persons with dementia actively practising social inclusion by being welcoming and supportive of their peers and visitors to the organization, including the researchers. As a testament to the inclusive environment created within the community organization, Motta-Ochoa et al. (2021) noted that individuals living with dementia were proud to share with their caregivers what they did at the activity centre to demonstrate that they were involved in meaningful and joyful activities with a social group that valued them.

Another example of how inclusive leisure environments contribute to reciprocal social experiences can be found in Robertson et al.'s (2020) study of inclusive walking groups, which consist of people with dementia and carers walking alongside the wider local population. Walking groups provided people living with dementia with opportunities to interact with a more diverse group than they otherwise would, supporting continued connections. The groups also provided people living with dementia with opportunities to offer support within the group by looking out for other participants. These findings highlighted how a supportive, inclusive walking group can help people living with dementia participate in their local community and maintain continued social participation – ultimately providing a space for social citizenship and for new social relationships to flourish.

Phinney et al.'s (2016) study of a community-based club for people living with young onset dementia provides another example of how daily walks in the neighbourhood can contribute to community connections and belonging. This study found that since participants viewed walking as an enjoyable pastime among a group of friends (rather than as a programme), and because it was something everyone could be part of, it took the focus away from participants' dementia. Intentional efforts by leaders to 'leave the diagnosis at the door' meant members could have fun and engage with what was happening around them. Since the primary aim of the club was for everyone to share in a meaningful and enjoyable activity, the act of walking in the neighbourhood together contributed to developing emotional connections and a sense of belonging. Phinney et al. (2016) also noted that walking in the neighbourhood gave people living with dementia the opportunity to engage with and contribute to their community – key aspects of social citizenship. For example, while walking, members mingled with neighbours and interacted with their neighbours' dogs, which enabled them to assume roles as friendly neighbours who contribute to their community in positive ways.

Each example outlined above depicts ways people living with dementia are engaging in acts of social citizenship and resisting stigma through their leisure. They do this by continuing to sustain valued identities, engage in personally meaningful experiences and establish reciprocal social connections that lead to a sense of belonging. One way valued identities can be sustained is when leisure experiences enable people living with dementia to focus on their skills and abilities (Genoe 2009). Furthermore, key features of meaningful leisure experiences for people living with dementia include enjoyment, connection and belonging (Genoe 2009). Leisure also supports freedom of choice. These features are common among the examples provided in this chapter. Another important aspect of these examples is that family, friends, other individuals living with dementia and leisure providers play important roles in helping people living with dementia resist stigma by supporting their continued engagement in meaningful leisure experiences.

While there are reduced social opportunities for people living with dementia and while stigma can reduce leisure participation (Fortune and McKeown 2016; Norval et al. 2021), we can take hope from examples demonstrating the many different possibilities for continued leisure engagement that contribute to positive depictions of dementia. Drawing from these examples, we make recommendations below for how people living with dementia, their friends and care partners, and leisure service providers can resist dementia-related stigma in ways that support inclusion and social citizenship for people living with dementia.

Conclusion

While a diagnosis of dementia may be associated with negative attitudes that can impact well-being, life can continue to be meaningful following a diagnosis of dementia. Leisure provides opportunities to counter beliefs about dementia that focus on loss and decline. The freedom inherent in leisure allows room for people to engage in acts of citizenship that demonstrate remaining strengths and abilities, connect to their identities and experience belonging and hope. As we saw in Vignette 9.1, Cecelia experienced stigma after she was diagnosed with dementia and others questioned her capabilities. Experiences that people living with dementia may choose to engage in during their free time can serve as reminders that, rather than 'empty shells', they are valued and active citizens with knowledge, skills, interests and dreams for the future. In the final part of the vignette we saw how Cecelia used leisure to demonstrate her knowledge, skills and interests and to remind others that she is a person. Leisure service and healthcare providers can support people living with dementia by checking their preconceived notions about the condition, providing welcoming and supportive environments and encouraging service users to actively resist stigma if they so choose. Family members and friends can encourage their loved ones to participate in meaningful leisure, seek out inclusive environments for them to connect with others and support continued participation in community life as a way of upholding their social citizenship.

While we realize there is still a long way to go to rid society of misunderstandings and assumptions that lead to dementia-related stigma, we take hope from the examples highlighted in this chapter. Each example shows possibilities, not only for resisting stigma, but also for helping to ensure a diagnosis of dementia does not mean an end to meaningful leisure experiences that enhance a person's identity, enjoyment, belonging and citizenship. Social citizenship entails opportunities to grow and participate in community life (O'Connor et al. 2018), often the essence of meaningful leisure experiences. We look forward to the day when these examples are not exceptional, but commonplace leisure experiences for people living with dementia.

So what does this mean in practice?

For those supporting or enabling the involvement in leisure of people living with dementia

- Leisure experiences that bring meaning and joy to individuals living with dementia are important. Consideration should be given to how such experiences could be enabled and what modifications can be made to ensure leisure experiences are inclusive.
- Reflect on assumptions and steps that could be taken to challenge stigma and discrimination. Consider ways to support social citizenship for individuals living with dementia.
- Leisure service providers who recognize that leisure experiences enable people living with dementia to sustain valued identities, to engage in personally meaningful activities and to make friends and acquaintances leading to a sense of belonging can become allies in the work to resist stigma and support social citizenship. When leisure providers understand that, with some adjustments, there are a variety of leisure experiences available for people living with dementia to enjoy, they will continuously work towards meeting the leisure needs of people living with dementia and letting them know that they are valued members of the community.

For people living with dementia or their informal or family carers

- People living with dementia could communicate their leisure interests to their friends, family and leisure providers and collectively discuss what resources and supports would help them to maintain meaningful leisure experiences.
- People living with dementia may also benefit from mutual support provided from other individuals living with dementia since opportunities to engage in leisure in an accepting and supportive environment can help remove pressure to conform to others' expectations and put the emphasis more squarely on experiencing moments of joy. These opportunities may also help people living with dementia discover the many ways they can contribute to the enjoyment and well-being of others.
- Friends and care partners can seek ways to support people living with dementia to continue to engage in the leisure experiences they most enjoy. By appreciating the ways people living with dementia continue to derive meaning from leisure, friends and care partners will also continue to enjoy shared social experiences that are mutually rewarding. Focusing on strengths and abilities while supporting people who are living with dementia may provide opportunities for them to try new leisure activities, be active in their communities and/or sustain engagement in meaningful activities.
- The role a person's social network plays in ensuring they have opportunities for leisure opportunities is central to enabling affirmation of identity,

enhancement of belonging and sparking of joy. We ask readers to consider ways they can support the development and/or maintenance of a social network for individuals living with dementia.

References

Alzheimer Society of Canada (2017) *2017 Awareness Survey Executive Summary.* Available at: https://alzheimer.ca/sites/default/files/documents/2017_AWARENESS-SURVEY_EXECUTIVE_SUMMARY_0.pdf (accessed 17 June 2022).

Benbow, S.M. and Jolley, D. (2012) Dementia: Stigma and its effects, *Neurodegenerative Disease Management*, 2(2): 165–72.

Fortune, D. and McKeown, J. (2016) Sharing the journey: Exploring a social leisure program for persons with dementia and their spouses, *Leisure Sciences*, 38(4): 373–87.

Fortune, D., Whyte, C. and Genoe, R. (2021) The interplay between leisure, friendship, and dementia, *Dementia*, 20(6): 2041–56.

Genoe, M.R. (2009) Living with hope in the midst of change: The meaning of leisure within the context of dementia. Unpublished doctoral thesis, University of Waterloo, Ontario, Canada.

Genoe, M.R. and Whyte, C. (2015) Confronting ageism through therapeutic recreation practice, *Leisure/Loisir*, 39(2): 235–52.

Goffman, E. (1968) *Stigma: Notes on the Management of Spoiled Identity.* Harmondsworth: Penguin.

Isene, T.A., Thygesen, H., Danbolt, L.J. and Stifoss-Hanssen, H. (2022) Embodied meaning-making in the experiences and behaviours of persons with dementia, *Dementia*, 21(2): 442–56.

Kane, M. and Cook, L. (2013) *Dementia 2013: The Hidden Voice of Loneliness.* London: Alzheimer's Society. Available at: https://www.alzheimers.org.uk/sites/default/files/migrate/downloads/dementia_2013_the_hidden_voice_of_loneliness.pdf (accessed 5 September 2021).

Mitchell, G., Dupuis, S.L. and Kontos, P. (2013) Dementia discourse: From imposed suffering to knowing other-wise, *Journal of Applied Hermeneutics*, 5: 1–19.

Motta-Ochoa, R., Leibing, A., Bresba, P. et al. (2021) 'You're part of us and we're happy to have you here': Practices of social inclusion for persons with dementia, *Clinical Gerontologist*, 44(4): 470–81.

Noone, S. and Jenkins, N. (2018) Digging for dementia: Exploring the experience of community gardening from the perspectives of people with dementia, *Aging & Mental Health*, 22 (7): 881–8.

Norval, R.S., Henderson, F. and Whittam, G. (2021) Playing the long game: Exploring the phenomenon of dementia-friendly golf, *Dementia*, 20(8): 2867–75.

O'Connor, D., Mann, J. and Wiersma, E. (2018) Stigma, discrimination and agency: Diagnostic disclosure as an everyday practice shaping social citizenship, *Journal of Aging Studies*, 44: 45–51.

Phinney, A., Kelson, E., Baumbusch, J. et al. (2016) Walking in the neighbourhood: Performing social citizenship in dementia, *Dementia*, 15(3): 381–94.

Robertson, J.M., Gibson, G., Pemble, C. et al. (2020) 'It is part of belonging': Walking groups to promote social health amongst people living with dementia, *Social Inclusion*, 8(3): 113–22.

Sass, C., Surr, C. and Lozano-Sufrategui, L. (2021) Expressions of masculine identity through sports-based reminiscence: An ethnographic study with community-dwelling men with dementia, *Dementia*, 20(6): 2170–87.

Shaw, S.M. (2006) Resistance, in C. Rojek, S. Shaw and A. Veal (eds) *Handbook of Leisure Studies* (pp. 533–46). London: Palgrave Macmillan.

Swaffer, K. (2014) Dementia: Stigma, language, and dementia-friendly, *Dementia*, 13(6): 709–13.

Wearing, B. (1998) *Leisure and Feminist Theory*. London: Sage.

Realm Three

Place, places and spaces – their nature, use and meaning

10 Third places as leisure environments

Elaine C. Wiersma, Nisha Sutherland, Carlina Marchese, Lindsay Watt, Claire Linton and Bailey Vandorp

Summary

Creating dementia-friendly environments with opportunities for freedom is vital for people living with dementia. This chapter focuses on two programmes offered for people living with dementia in north-western Ontario, Canada: an art programme called *(re)Creating the Self* and a social programme called *Dementia Cafe: A Place to Belong*, with emphasis on the experiences of leisure and freedom. We consider both programmes as 'third places' for people living with dementia, their friends and their families. By 'third place' we mean an informal place in which people relax and socialize that is not their home or work. Third places can be used to create strong relationships between participants and a sense of community – for example, by organizing the environment so it feels like a home away from home, allowing people to be themselves. This chapter explores how both the social and the physical environments of the programmes contributed to the experiences of leisure described by participants. Leisure environments provide opportunities for people to experience freedom – both *freedom to be* and *freedom to do*. *Freedom to be* focuses on the opportunities that people felt they had to be themselves, be included and be connected with others. *Freedom to do* describes the freedom to create and express oneself, found in both programmes. In the chapter, we also discuss characteristics of both programmes showing how their physical and social environments influenced perceptions of freedom. For example:

- *freedom to be* – where people felt freedom from labels, judgement and worry
- *freedom to do* – where people felt able to participate in activities that promote self-expression without fear of failure.

When developing leisure programmes for people living with dementia and their families, the concept of third places should be considered, because these provide an important way to create a sense of community, inclusion and *freedom to be*.

Leisure, dementia and freedom

The meaning of leisure has been a subject of philosophy for as far back as Aristotle and his conceptualization of the good life (Mannell and Kleiber 1997). How each individual comprehends the leisure they take part in has been seen as fundamental in defining it (Harper 1986). However, the cognitive challenges people living with dementia experience, and the stigma associated with the condition, mean people living with dementia experience fewer opportunities to freely engage in leisure. When leisure is seen as a psychological state, the person living with dementia is viewed more as an individual with a debilitating cognitive condition, and less as a person with capabilities, preferences and with needs and aspirations to be an active citizen. Thus, rather than emphasizing leisure as solely a state of mind, it is vital to pay attention to the physical, social and political environments in which people living with dementia feel free to be (i.e. be themselves) and do (i.e. do activities or be creative) (Hemingway 1996).

For people living with dementia, leisure provides opportunities to live and experience life to the fullest, despite the diagnosis of dementia (Dupuis et al. 2012). After a diagnosis, people living with dementia and their care partners use strategies to maintain their engagement with leisure (Fortune et al. 2021) and adapt to sustain their friendships with others (Genoe et al. 2021). While dementia can pose challenges to such engagement, leisure can play a role in finding hope and meaning in life (Genoe and Dupuis 2014). Leisure is at the centre of shared experiences for people living with dementia and their friends (Fortune et al. 2021) and can take many forms, including those of arts-based activities or social activities involving valued social connections that can be built within certain settings, including those informal spaces sometimes termed 'third places' (Oldenburg 1999) in which people relax and socialize away from home or work.

The purpose of this chapter is to describe leisure as freedom for people living with dementia, using the examples of two programmes – an art programme and a Dementia Cafe social programme – and to examine how physical and social environments influence perceptions of freedom.

Arts-based activities

Arts-based activities as leisure may include visual arts, music, dance, singing and literary arts. These can be inexpensive and accessible as they can include all senses and can be undertaken without prior knowledge and despite memory loss. Moreover, art can promote socialization and a sense of belonging for people living with dementia (Schneider 2018). A variety of positive outcomes linked to participation in arts-based activity for people living with dementia include providing a calming effect, a personal sense of control and helping to ameliorate behavioural and emotional changes (Cowl and Gaugler 2014). Beyond enjoyment, arts-based programming has been reported to improve quality of life, increase well-being and self-esteem and promote a sense of inclusion. It has been shown that the arts benefit not only the person living with dementia, but also care partners, by contributing to enhanced cultural capital (Schneider 2018).

Social connections

Social connections are important components of recreational activities, particularly when these take place in group settings. Being sociable, especially with one's peers, enables new relationships and friendships with other people living with dementia (Dupuis and Gillies 2014; Keyes et al. 2014). Groups for people living with dementia afford benefits, like providing a place of belonging (Ward et al. 2012), sharing common experiences, offering a place of safety where people do not have to be embarrassed about their limitations (Ward et al. 2012; Dupuis and Gillies 2014) and providing opportunities to share information about coping with changes related to dementia (Ward et al. 2012; Keyes et al. 2014). These social connections typically take place in built environments and third places.

Third places

As detailed above, a third place is an informal and inclusive public space where a person may enjoy casual socialization when not at home or work (Oldenburg 1999). Third places may be coffee shops, bookstores, bars, hair salons or other places where people get together. They are considered neutral, where everyone is welcome and equal in the space, with a casual feel, where the environment is light-hearted, and where conversation is the focus, allowing social connections to be formed.

Third places are important contributors to age-friendly communities and can enhance the health and well-being of older people as they engage in the social life of their community (Alidoust et al. 2019). Older adults who regularly access a third place are more likely to enjoy better health and well-being (Cheang 2002), a means of gaining social capital and empowerment (Meshram and O'Cass 2013) and emotional support (Fong et al. 2021). Third places may offer some reprieve from the loneliness associated with loss of social support from bereavement, retirement or other major life events that are more likely to impact older adults (Rosenbaum et al. 2007).

However, third places should not be accepted as exclusively positive. For example, older adults can face barriers to third places, such as changes in health, mobility and driving ability (Alidoust et al. 2019) as well as stigma. Third places might never be a neutral space because of overarching gender, status or race power relations likely remaining present within any societal context (Soukup 2006; Yuen and Johnson 2017). Social inclusion might be a better goal for third places rather than accessibility, as some places and activities currently may be welcome to some, but not to others (Yuen and Johnson 2017).

In summary, leisure has been conceptualized as a state of mind rather than solely an activity. Extensive benefits of leisure have been outlined, particularly of perceived freedom. However, how the physical and social environments facilitate or create opportunities for perceived freedom for people living with dementia, and the impact of environmental factors, need to be better understood. It is to this we now turn, using two programmes offered for people living with dementia as illustrative examples.

Leisure environments for people living with dementia

The *(re)Creating the Self* art programme, based in north-western Ontario, was developed in partnership with a local non-profit organization, the local art gallery and an academic institution. Each programme was four weeks long, consisting of two-hour sessions once a week facilitated by a local artist at an art gallery. In the related research project on which we report here, data were collected from three programmes over the course of one year. The participants, who were living with dementia, created collective pieces of art including a paper quilt, a banner and a large book. All were over the age of 65 and had been diagnosed within the last five to ten years. Some individuals participated in more than one programme. The collective artwork was displayed in public community spaces and was put together by the participants who helped choose the photographs of the art.

Data collection included participant observations conducted during the programme, as well as a debriefing period of up to 15 minutes conducted at the end of each group session. During this time, participants were asked questions such as 'What did you like about today? What surprised you? What challenged you?'. Additionally, photographs taken during the sessions focused on participant interactions, activities and engagement with the art materials and art pieces. A reflective group celebration was held with two care partners and four participants, as well as a final focus group with the artist facilitator and two other group supporters. Participants were invited to help write a book chapter which has previously reported on the findings (Wiersma et al. 2019).

The second programme, *Dementia Cafe: A Place to Belong* (hereafter referred to as Dementia Cafe), is a social venture that offers a safe and inclusive environment for people living with dementia and their family and friends. Dementia Cafe provides attendees with opportunities for social interaction and connections that help to decrease isolation, and informational resources. Dementia Cafe began in 2018 and is a partnership between the Centre for Education and Research on Aging & Health at Lakehead University and Urban Abbey. The programme runs on Sunday afternoons at Urban Abbey, which is a reclaimed old church that has been reconstituted as a modern-day Celtic abbey. Volunteers assist in a variety of roles and are all people living with dementia and their care partners. Dementia Cafe is run by Elaine Wiersma and two part-time staff who provide logistical and administrative support.

Ten Dementia Cafe participants were interviewed for the study: two people living with dementia, five family members and three people acting as volunteers within the programme. A semi-structured interview guide was used to explore the participants' experiences of Dementia Cafe, including the benefits, social interactions, space and any improvements. The audio-recorded interviews were then transcribed and analysed for themes.

The analysis of these two programmes showed that participants described their experiences with reference to two key elements: *freedom to be* and *freedom to do*. *Freedom to be* focused on the opportunities that people felt they experienced to be themselves, to be included and to be with others. *Freedom to do* described the freedom to create and the freedom to express oneself found in both programmes. *Freedom to be* was found to be a necessary precursor for *freedom to do*. The environment, both physical and social, played a role in creating these spaces of freedom. Findings are presented here as overall themes since commonalities were found among the experiences of participants in the two programmes.

Freedom to be

Three themes emerged: free to be ourselves, free to belong and free to be relational.

Free to be ourselves

In the art programme, participants talked about the opportunity to be themselves, including not having to cover up any dementia-related limitations. For example, Abigail stated, 'You don't have to be afraid of saying or expressing something.' Hilary said, 'We look forward to coming and being ourselves.' Laura related, 'It's nice to be able to forget about it [dementia] and not to feel so alone.'

At the Dementia Cafe, people living with dementia felt free 'to be' themselves. Being there meant freedom from labels, judgement and worry. Joanne said:

> nobody's there to judge you … or wait for you to make a mistake or say something wrong … Like I don't remember some things and I should remember them maybe. But with the Alzheimer's and that, you forget. So there, when you're in that group, you don't have to worry about remembering to say Mary Lou is her name or something like that, you know. Do you get what I mean? [laughter].

Family members witnessed how the environment at the Dementia Cafe was contributing to a safe space in which their relatives with dementia could freely express themselves. As Leah, an adult daughter, noted:

> So they [people living with dementia] know that decline is happening. And they try to hide it, right? They try to hide that they're not okay. And so, I would just stress that it's okay. You can be who you are. It's okay if your hands are tremoring or – nobody cares. Everybody just – will be happy to see you and welcome you to the community.

Free to belong

While the goal of the art programme was not necessarily belonging, participants described feeling like they were included and belonged. This was typically described as feeling 'comfortable' in the programme and with other participants, despite the fact that many were initially hesitant about the programme. As Barbara said, 'You just feel comfortable as though you belong here and that you belong with people, so that you can sort of take that to the community and be with people and still be yourself, without being too self-conscious about your problems and hold everything back in.' Other participants described how comfortable they felt. As Edward related, 'For me it's – I feel comfortable and I enjoy what I'm doing.'

The goal of *Dementia Cafe: A Place to Belong*, as indicated in its title, is to create a place of belonging for participants. Many described that feeling of belonging. A large part of this was enabled through connecting with other people and being included in conversations. Donald, who is living with dementia stated: 'Connected, happy, those two words probably sum it up more than anything. Connected from the standpoint that you can get into some really, really good conversations. And I think if you connect with people, the happiness aspect comes secondary to that.' An adult daughter, Leah, also described the feeling of belonging: 'Oh, everybody is so nice and so kind and so understanding and, you know, so receiving of people, the way life is supposed to be, like, that unconditional love, do no harm, heart centred, yeah, yeah. And it's so wonderful, we feel like we belong. They help us feel like we belong.'

Freedom to be relational

Both the art programme and Dementia Cafe created environments where people were free to be relational (i.e. be with others) and create new friendships. In reflecting on their experiences in the art programme, participants described the friendships they created. As Samantha stated, 'We're all a bunch of sisters ... these are my new buddies, whether they like it or not [laughter].' Barbara also said: 'The people I have met have been wonderful. Wonderful camaraderie. We can have fun and laugh and make fun of ourselves.'

At Dementia Cafe, people living with dementia and their care partners attended primarily to be with friends. As James, a family care partner said: 'You don't even think about where you are. You think you're just going to meet a bunch of friends. You're not going to a venue of dementia or Alzheimer's and all that. You look forward to going to meet the people you've made friends with.'

Donald, a person living with dementia, described the feeling of family created at Dementia Cafe: 'It's like a giant family. Again, some of the people who come, particularly the ones who are coming at the present time ... but it's like a big family gathering ... From the moment you walk in, everybody is friendly. It's a case of, "What can we do for you today?" It's just a big family gathering.'

And James, the husband and care partner of a woman living with dementia, elaborated further:

It seems every Cafe we meet somebody new, and of course you see them walk in. They're a little bit shy and hesitant and you walk up to them and strike up a conversation and try and make them feel at home too. Feel comfortable where we're at. It's just, it's an amazing experience that we are in a room where we can feel comfortable with not a very nice situation, but it makes it one of the things that makes it easier to accept that there's a facility like this and people that you get to meet.

Freedom to do

Creating an environment that enabled freedom to be oneself, to be included and to be relational was critical for participants to experience *freedom to do*. We characterize *freedom to do* as the freedom to participate in activities both in the art programme and at Dementia Cafe without fear. We do not conceptualize this as failure-free activity because the very notion of failure indicates that someone's creation is either a success or a failure. Rather, we see *freedom to do* as freedom to participate in activities that promote self-expression without fear of failure. There is no failure or success, rather, just an opportunity to express oneself through activity. There were two components of *freedom to do* – freedom to create and freedom to express.

Freedom to create

Participants described how they felt free to create. A number were hesitant to join the art programme because they had preconceived ideas of what they thought art was. Lillian said: 'Art is a little different than I thought it was. It's kind of nice to know [laughter]. I didn't realize I just [thought] – drawing is art – that's it. I found out different things. Everything is art.' And, as Laura stated: '… see how creative we were. Who knew? It kind of made us stretch. I mean we had to use our ingenuity to try to incorporate this for us, you know? It was good. Everybody did something different too.'

Freedom to express

Part of the creative process is expressing oneself through the medium available. In the case of the art programme, participants described the opportunity and ability to express themselves through the art activities. Hilary stated, '… it just brings out in you that you do have some imagination and you can do certain things and nobody's going to say anything about it because everybody just puts their own into it and I think it's fantastic'. As part of that expression, there was no expectation of perfection. Daniel said: 'I enjoyed the idea of knowing that it doesn't have to be perfect. It's close enough.' Indeed, any type of creative self-expression does not have success standards, since the expression of oneself is the goal. As Hilary stated: 'You can't make a mess. You can't screw it up. Who's going to say – "You should've done…"?'

At Dementia Cafe, people living with dementia and their partners also felt the freedom to express themselves through dance, singing or just being silly.

Leah, the daughter of a man living with dementia, stated: 'When they have dance day or something, we'd get up and we'd both be dancing, and he'd be clapping, and everybody got a kick out of that. They were like, oh, look at [name] and then I, you know, grab his arms or, you know, just silly, silly things … Just act silly, it doesn't matter how old you are, you can act silly.'

An adult daughter, Jolene, recounted how singing and dancing allowed her mother, who lives with dementia, to express her feelings and created a special relational bond:

> So, with being able to dance with my mother and we'll sing with each other when we're dancing. And my mom never was a person who would tell you she loved you or anything like that or, you know, she was very closed, and so it was very special [crying] … the last dance we danced was, 'I can't help falling in love with you', and she was singing to me.

Place as an enabler of freedom

The physical environment

Earlier, we introduced third places and suggested that not every third place will be inclusive of people living with dementia. Chloe, a volunteer for Dementia Café, commented on this and suggested why remedying it is important:

> Because again, going back to those that are living the road, walking the road and living the space of being, coping with dementia, their world has changed dramatically and continues to change hourly, weekly, whatever. So absolutely, I think that having a third place as someone living with dementia or someone caring with dementia is so important because so many of those other spaces and places have become out of reach or closed off to them.

The art programme was held in a community room at the local art gallery – a public space accessible to the community. Participants were able to browse the galleries. Several participants commented on how being able to use the physical space contributed to the *freedom to be* and *freedom to do*. Barbara related: 'I liked it too [going into the art gallery]. I like to enjoy it and come and go in there other times too.' The space in the community room had a large window looking out to the forest which also had some outdoor sculptures. Daniel said: 'See that tree out there with all the snow on it. I mean, that would make a good picture to show them to say our art and craft or something like that. Just you know, with the sun on it, everything showing up just perfect.'

Edward also commented on how the art gallery was the ideal setting for the programme, saying, 'I found that interesting while we're in an appropriate setting to do that – to be creative.'

Dementia Cafe is held in a historic church with pews removed. It has a very high ceiling, large stained-glass windows and a coffee shop attached. The history of the church, its current use and the unique space gave participants a sense of comfort and peace, as described by Olivia, a volunteer:

> So, you kind of feel a natural sense of being at peace when you go into the building and the windows are just beautiful when the sun comes in with the white walls. It gives a nice reflection which is very colourful. So, colours as well as the acoustics for just being able to speak to one another, it's, you get this feeling ... you have a sense of belonging ... a sense of peace.

Joanne, a person living with dementia, commented on how the old church gave a feeling like coming home:

> Like it's homey. Like you know, it's comfortable there ... It's a good mix with whatever's going ... it all fits ... Like whoever set it up ... it's done amazingly. I've seen people come in there and be kind of quiet and not say much or whatever, and the first thing you know, the next time we saw them, they were chatting with people and everything. So, it's the atmosphere that comes from the people and the place that we're in.

Several other participants commented on how the environment was home-like, despite the very large space of the church, which was quite unlike a home. These feelings of comfort, peace and home-like attest to the fit of the physical and social environment, and the vital role the environment plays in creating a programme that allows people the freedom to be and do.

The social environment, also characteristic of third places, was critical to experiencing freedom as well. The participants described the supporters and volunteers of both programmes as essential to this freedom. Barbara said, of the volunteers and facilitators of the art programme: 'And you people have been really, really excellent with all of us. I think you've met us all as a friend rather than someplace that maybe you just don't want to come to and I think we've learned a lot and I think that we all – we can do something else together and keep it going.'

Abigail stated, 'I would say knowing that the people that we work with – with you guys – makes us comfortable enough to be doing a lot of things.' A family member, Hazel, expressed that in addition to the nonjudgemental atmosphere provided, the volunteers at Dementia Cafe treated her father with respect and dignity: 'At Dementia Cafe they are seen as wise people who have lived full lives and so people are treated respectfully. And again, that comes back to even using their names and engaging with them and being understanding of their condition.'

This *freedom to be* was critical for people to feel included and was further accomplished through activities that provided opportunities for people living with dementia to contribute to fun social interactions.

Volunteers also stated the importance of people living with dementia and care partners feeling comfortable and free to mingle with others. One volunteer, Olivia, commented on how the name tags were helpful in allowing the meeting of and socializing with strangers:

> Well, I like the way that it's set up where everyone comes in and regardless of the fact that you're a volunteer or you're a visitor you all have the same

name tag on and it's just your first name. So you get to know each other that way ... because you have your name tags on, everybody does know each other, so you don't feel that oh, well, 'that person over there knows that one, I'm just going to sit here by myself'.

The name tags gave a sense of equality for all involved, affording a sense of freedom and comfort to 'be'. Olivia added: 'Everyone has a name tag on. We're all the same, which is how it should be.' The feeling that everyone was seen as equals meant that people living with dementia and their care partners were included in participation.

Conclusion – using leisure environments to promote freedom

In this chapter we have sought to show how two different leisure environments for people living with dementia were used, and how, across both environments, this use enabled those participating to experience *freedom to be* and *freedom to do*. Consistent with literature in leisure studies, freedom was a critical component of these two programmes for people living with dementia. Freedom was reflected both in individual states and perceptions, as well as issues relating more broadly to society and culture which were shown in participants' comments.

People living with dementia and care partners talked about a freedom to be themselves. The finding of a freedom to be oneself indicates the difficulty, discomfort and stigma that many people living with dementia experience in everyday life (Wiersma et al. 2016) and the feeling of safety and freedom that comes with leisure environments used in the ways we have described. People living with dementia repeatedly emphasized the importance of being able to be oneself, to not worry about needing to maintain a mask of normalcy, nor worry about how others view the cognitive challenges that accompany dementia. The art programme and Dementia Cafe environments provided a reprieve from some adverse features common to everyday life for people living with dementia and their families, particularly the reactions of others that feel stigmatizing.

These leisure environments also provided opportunities for inclusion that were contrary to the more familiar experience of exclusion. Indeed, other studies have suggested that creating environments for people living with dementia to connect with each other should be prioritized (Wiersma et al. 2016; Fortune et al. 2021). Third places act as a leveller – meaning that everyone is welcome and equal in the space. The comments of participants about Dementia Cafe demonstrate that this was a space where people felt equal. With the art programme, the social and physical structure of that environment created a space where participants felt pride in their accomplishments and where they described themselves as artists and as creative.

We note the similarities between our findings and many of the characteristics of third places. Third places have a casual atmosphere, and both programmes offered this. Participants talked about the lack of expectation and worry about their cognitive challenges with dementia because others were also experiencing the same thing. Third places can also be seen as a home away from home, allowing people to be themselves. That leisure environments can be used to enable this is a key finding. We suggest that these leisure environments, and by extension other leisure environments, can be considered third places and have an important role to play in creating a sense of community for people living with dementia and their families.

We recognize that there are differences between the programmes and more established interpretations of third places. First, a characteristic of third places is that they are on neutral ground, where no one assumes the role of host. Since the art programme includes a facilitator, this characteristic may not specifically apply. In addition, at Dementia Cafe, volunteers act as table hosts, helping to facilitate conversation when necessary. Second, a third place has conversation as the main activity. While conversation was an important part of the art programme, it was not a stated goal. Dementia Cafe, on the other hand, had social interaction and conversation as primary activities.

The concept of third places should be used to better understand the ways in which leisure programmes and environments can provide opportunities for freedom for people living with dementia and their families. While structured programmes (such as the art programme) are important for people's well-being, the need for casual social programmes is also important. Using the example of Dementia Cafe, we suggest that there is a requirement for more places, open for longer hours, in which people living with dementia and their families can socialize and find opportunities to be themselves.

Leisure environments provide opportunities for people to experience freedom—both *freedom to be* and *freedom to do*. Physical and social environments are critical to providing opportunities for this. The concept of third places should be used when developing leisure programmes for people living with dementia and their families as an important way to create a sense of community, inclusion and freedom.

So what does this mean in practice?

For those supporting or enabling the involvement in leisure of people living with dementia

- *Freedom to be* is an essential precursor of the *freedom to do*.
- The physical environment should facilitate comfort, connection and inclusion to ensure people feel free to belong.
- The social environment should allow people living with dementia to be free to be themselves, with a sense of equality, without labels, judgement or worry.

For people living with dementia or their informal or family carers

- Feelings of inclusion and belonging are important aspects of leisure programmes.
- Third spaces and leisure programmes provide environments to develop and nurture friendship and comradery.
- People living with dementia and their carers may experience the freedom to be themselves around others who share their lived experiences.

For researchers

- Further research is required to better understand how leisure programmes and environments can create *freedom to be* and *freedom to do* for people living with dementia and their carers.
- Additional research is needed on the physical characteristics of leisure environments that can facilitate positive experiences and nurture relationships.
- Further research is needed on the role of supporters in creating and facilitating physical and social environments for people with dementia and their carers.

References

Alidoust, S., Bosman, C. and Holden, G. (2019) Planning for healthy ageing: How the use of third places contributes to the social health of older populations, *Ageing and Society*, 39(7): 1459–84.

Cheang, M. (2002) Older adult's frequent visits to a fast-food restaurant: Nonobligatory social interaction and the significance of play in a 'third place', *Journal of Aging Studies*, 16(3): 303–21.

Cowl, A.L. and Gaugler, J.E. (2014) Efficacy of creative arts therapy in treatment of Alzheimer's disease and dementia: A systematic literature review, *Activities, Adaptation and Aging*, 38(4): 281–330.

Dupuis, S.L. and Gillies, J. (2014) Learning as a vehicle for individual and social transformation: Re-thinking leisure education, *Therapeutic Recreation Journal*, 48(2): 113–34.

Dupuis, S.L., Whyte, C., Carson, J. et al. (2012) Just dance with me: An authentic partnership approach to understanding leisure in the dementia context, *World Leisure Journal*, 54(3): 240–54.

Fong, P., Haslam, C., Cruwys, T. and Haslam, S.A. (2021) 'There's a bit of a ripple-effect': A social identity perspective on the role of third-places and aging in place, *Environment and Behavior*, 53(5): 540–68.

Fortune, D., Whyte, C. and Genoe, R. (2021) The interplay between leisure, friendship, and dementia, *Dementia*, 20(6): 2041–56.

Genoe, M.R. and Dupuis, S.L. (2014) The role of leisure within the dementia context, *Dementia*, 13(1): 33–58.

Genoe, M.R., Fortune, D. and Whyte, C. (2021) Strategies for maintaining friendship in dementia, *Canadian Journal on Aging*, 41(3): 1–12.

Harper, W. (1986) Freedom in the experience of leisure, *Leisure Sciences*, 8(2): 115–30.

Hemingway, J.L. (1996) Emancipating leisure: The recovery of freedom in leisure, *Journal of Leisure Research*, 28(1): 27–43.

Keyes, S.E., Clarke, C.L., Wilkinson, H. et al. (2014) 'We're all thrown in the same boat …': A qualitative analysis of peer support in dementia care, *Dementia*, 5(4): 560–77.

Mannell, R.C. and Kleiber, D.A. (1997) *A Social Psychology of Leisure*. Champaign, IL: Venture Publishing.

Meshram, K. and O'Cass, A. (2013) Empowering senior citizens via third places: Research driven model development of seniors' empowerment and social engagement in social places, *Journal of Services Marketing*, 27(2): 141–54.

Oldenburg, R. (1999) *The Great Good Place: Cafes, Coffee Shops, Bookstores, Bars, Hair Salons, and Other Hangouts at the Heart of a Community*, 2nd edn. New York: Da Capo Press.

Rosenbaum, M.S., Ward, J., Walker, B.A. et al. (2007) A cup of coffee with a dash of love: An investigation of commercial social support and third-place attachment, *Journal of Service Research*, 10(1): 43–59.

Schneider, J. (2018) The arts as a medium for care and self-care in dementia: Arguments and evidence, *International Journal of Environmental Research and Public Health*, 15(6): 1151.

Soukup, C. (2006) Computer-mediated communication as a virtual third place: Building Oldenburg's great good places on the world wide web, *New Media and Society*, 8(3): 421–40.

Ward, R., Howorth, M., Wilkinson, H. et al. (2012) Supporting the friendships of people with dementia, *Dementia*, 11(3): 287–303.

Wiersma, E.C., Berry, J., Glover, J. et al. (2019) Art as the great equalizer: Everyday citizenship and participation in an art program for people with dementia, in A.C. Nedlund, R. Bartlett and C. Clarke (eds) *Everyday Citizenship and People with Dementia*. Edinburgh: Dunedin Press.

Wiersma, E.C., O'Connor, D., Loiselle, L. et al. (2016) Creating space for citizenship: The impact of group structure on validating the voices of people with dementia, *Dementia*, 15(3): 414–33.

Yuen, F. and Johnson, A.J. (2017) Leisure spaces, community, and third places, *Leisure Sciences*, 39(3): 295–303.

Connecting with nature

Simon Evans

Summary

Humans have an innate connection with the outdoors, and the famous psychiatrist Carl Jung described the natural world as 'the nourishing soil of the soul'. The pressures of modern life, a greater focus on mental health, and Covid-19 have driven an interest in the benefits of getting outdoors and connecting with nature. This can be seen in various initiatives such as mindfulness and forest bathing. Evidence highlights the benefits of getting outdoors and connecting with nature for people living with dementia, including improved physical and mental health, better sleep patterns, greater levels of social interaction and feelings of happiness. Going for a walk, doing some gardening and putting out food for birds are all good examples of popular outdoor activities. Enjoying connections with nature may be enough for some people living with dementia, but it is also important to have opportunities to engage in outdoor leisure activities which have meaning, can support a sense of identity and allow someone to contribute to their community or neighbourhood. However, many people living with dementia face challenges to getting outdoors, particularly in some care settings. This is often because of attitudes towards dementia, gardens that are difficult to access and misunderstandings about the benefits and risks related to outdoor environments. The research presented in this chapter highlights ways of overcoming the challenges. These include making sure surfaces are flat and easy to walk on/use with a wheelchair, having clarity about how people living with dementia can play a role in the outdoor space (for example, contribute to gardening), or even bringing the outdoors inside by, for example, making plants and picked flowers available if going outside is impossible.

Introduction

This chapter draws on research that I undertook in the UK to explore the various benefits for people living with dementia of connecting with nature and getting outdoors, highlighting the role leisure activities can play. It also looks at some of the challenges that prevent people from getting outdoors, along with some of the solutions. I conclude that having opportunities to connect with nature, both inside and outdoors, should be seen as a key element of inclusive citizenship and a basic human right, not just a nice day out.

The advantages of connecting with nature

The concept of 'biophilia' suggests that interaction with nature is essential to our psychological health (Wilson 1984). Similarly, environmental psychologists have suggested that the natural environment addresses an innate need for contemplation, restoration and distraction (Kaplan 1995). A growing body of research evidence indicates that connecting with nature is closely associated with quality of life, mental health and well-being (Mensah et al. 2016). An increasing interest in the health-related or 'salutogenic' benefits of nature is reflected in contemporary movements such as mindfulness (purposely bringing one's attention in the present moment), biophilic cities and forest bathing – a Japanese process of relaxation through the simple method of being calm and quiet among the trees (Lee et al. 2011). Numerous studies have identified benefits of connecting with nature for older people in general, including reduced anxiety, improved sleep and increased happiness (Barrett et al. 2019). People living with dementia may gain from improved eating patterns, better mood, reduced agitation, positive reminiscence and even enhanced cognition (Motealleh et al. 2019). It has been suggested that some of the positive impacts of connecting with nature are associated with increased opportunities for social interaction, increased independence and maintaining specific outdoor hobbies and activities (Hendriks et al. 2016). Opportunities of this sort are intrinsically associated with the concepts of leisure and social citizenship as explored in this chapter.

Ways of connecting with nature

While there is a myriad of ways to connect with nature, much of the research has focused on specific settings. For example, a study of 'green care' in nine extra care housing schemes and care homes in England found that opportunities to connect with nature often came from leisure-based pastimes such as walking and gardening (Evans et al. 2019). Other popular nature-based activities were trips to scenic locations, walking in the countryside and having contact with animals that lived in the scheme or were brought in for that specific purpose. For some people in the study who rarely went outdoors, the main connection with nature occurred indoors, through activities including arts and crafts, bird-watching through the window and nature programmes on television. One member of staff described the impact of bringing the outdoors in as follows: 'I can take a basketful of flowers I picked outside, roses and stuff like that, and take them to people to smell and their eyes open, that may be the first time I've seen their eyes open for weeks, you know, so it's still worth it.'

There were also several examples of animals being brought indoors for residents to enjoy, including guinea pigs, rabbits and dogs. One case study site in this research was a care home that incorporated a 'pet farm', where participants were able to help look after and handle a range of animals including goats, ducks, parrots and fish. There were many examples of the enjoyment that contact with these animals brought, with one resident saying 'I try to give them a bit of food … have a chat to them. They don't answer, though the parrots do occasionally.' An activity coordinator employed at the home felt that the farm brought benefits to residents: 'The animals have a massive impact because it's giving them a purpose every single day. It's giving them something to look after. It's giving them responsibility again.' This links with the idea of communicative leisure (Spracklen 2013), whereby leisure activities are seen as a fundamental part of our humanity, helping to shape who we are and enabling individuals to forge meaning in relation to identity and their place in the world.

Many care settings have established sensory gardens with the aim of promoting well-being for people living with dementia. This approach incorporates the use of surfaces, objects and plants that stimulate senses through touch, sight, scent, taste and hearing. There is some evidence for their positive health benefits, including a reduction in serious falls, improved sleep patterns and reduced prescribing of medication used to treat mental health disorders (Gonzalez and Kirkevold 2015).

In 2020 a project was carried out in England by a social enterprise organization with the aim of increasing opportunities and choices for people living with dementia, largely by supporting their involvement in outdoor activities. This project provided training and support for staff at four national organizations offering care and/or support to people living with dementia to encourage the delivery of a wide range of nature-based activities to participants. These activities included farming, but also leisure pursuits such as gardening, visits to the beach, flower arranging and interacting with animals. Findings from the research accompanying the project suggested that taking part in activities was associated with statistically significant increases in self-reported well-being for people living with dementia and their family carers (Evans et al. 2021). People living with dementia also reported statistically significant increases in their weekly levels of physical activity. However, it is of equal importance that these activities increased opportunities and choices for participants.

Case study sites in the research included: a care farm providing support for people affected by dementia through involvement in a range of hands-on farming activities, including planting, fruit and vegetable cultivation, helping to restore farm buildings, animal husbandry and the basics of machinery maintenance; a care home where two activity coordinators provided a programme of inclusive activities including quizzes, gentle exercise classes and outings to local attractions; and an organization providing intergenerational, craft-based activities in a woodland, with a focus on being outdoors and socializing, especially between generations, in order to improve mental health and well-being. People living with dementia who took part in the research spoke about their past lives and explained that they still considered themselves to be capable, skilled people. The project helped them to reconnect with their earlier lives and identities through activities such as farming and cooking. Staff suggested that undertaking 'real' tasks was fulfilling for participants, although the importance of not asking too much of those living with dementia was also stressed. This suggests that connecting with nature might provide opportunities for people living with dementia to engage in leisure activities.

One participant, Peter, had a career as a chef before developing dementia. By attending the care farm, he had the opportunity to pursue his continuing skills and interests by helping to prepare the lunch that was provided. Peter's family carer recognized the enjoyment that this gave him, saying: 'He used to be a chef, and a lot of the time they let him in the kitchen, and he makes soup so all the people who are there that day, they all have soup and a bread roll for lunch.' A member of staff from a care home participating in the project described how outdoor activities impacted on one of the residents: 'John came alive in the gardens, remembering his wife's garden and saying how proud he was of her.' Another staff member recalled how, on a boat trip that was arranged for a group of residents, one man called Rupert and his wife enjoyed 'giggling on a date together'. He felt that this experience had allowed them to be a couple again, instead of being seen as a carer and person to be cared for, providing a clear example of how leisure activities can promote social citizenship by enabling someone to sustain their place in everyday life (Nedlund et al. 2019).

For most people living with dementia, being in their own garden or local neighbourhood will provide the best opportunity for connecting with nature on a regular basis. A study exploring the role of gardens in the everyday lives of people living with dementia at home during the Covid-19 pandemic found that gardens provided a sense of enjoyment and empowerment (Buse and Balmer 2021). They were specifically valued as a sensory experience, for being 'in the moment', and triggering enjoyable memories. Gardens also facilitated social interaction, not just with family and friends but also with neighbours over boundary fences and walls. Participants would often sit outdoors with a cup of tea or coffee or spend mealtimes outside when the weather was good enough. This highlights the value of incorporating garden use into daily routines, as well as the need for seating that is well placed and sufficiently comfortable. Having a good view of the garden from indoors was also important because it enabled a connection with nature when the weather was not good enough be outside. While in many ways Covid-19 has had a particularly harsh impact on people living with dementia, it has also given insight into the experience of having limited opportunities to enjoy leisure activities and the social interaction that they can provide.

Designing outdoor places for leisure activities

A review of the literature published in 2021 highlighted the importance of design for people living with dementia across a range of environments, including outdoor spaces (Evans et al. 2021). This is largely because Alzheimer's disease and many other dementias result in significant declines in navigation skills, which can be exacerbated when someone moves to an unfamiliar environment such as a care home. The authors identified five things that should be considered in the design of the built environment, both indoors and outdoors:

- *Meaningful activity* – leisure, physical, social and activities tailored to the person's needs and preferences.
- *Legibility* – spaces that make their purpose clear and obvious and allow people to see and find each other.
- *Orientation* – a sense of time and place.
- *Wayfinding* – the ability to navigate a space.
- *Familiarity* – maximizing the value of someone's existing knowledge and experience.

Careful consideration of these domains by those who plan, design, manage and advocate for outdoor places can help promote for people living with dementia easier decision-making, reduced agitation and distress, increased independence and social interaction, enhanced safety and the ability to carry out everyday tasks.

Dementia-friendly design principles have received much attention in recent years, including the development of various tools that aim to support such work. Suggestions for maximizing the use of domestic gardens include placing a comfortable chair in a quiet sheltered area where someone can rest, removing any planting that is poisonous, irritant to the skin or has thorns, and using signage or a landmark as a reminder of how to get back into the house and the toilet.[1]

How to support connections with nature

Despite growing recognition of the substantial benefits of connections with nature for people living with dementia, many outdoor spaces remain underused. There are numerous reasons for this: access may be difficult, particularly in bad weather, or the space may look uncared for or be felt to be unsafe due to poor maintenance. Access can be particularly challenging for people with impaired mobility or sight, especially when there are potential safety hazards such as steps or uneven surfaces. There are often challenges to easy access to outdoor spaces in some care settings. The 'green care' study mentioned above reported a wide range of barriers to getting outdoors and connecting with nature. The design of the physical environment was most commonly cited, both in terms of barriers accessing the garden and in relation to difficulties getting around once in it. In many care homes people living with dementia are supported in a separate area, often on an upper floor. This can severely limit opportunities to go outside, both as a planned activity and on a spontaneous basis. Even with good access to the outdoors, people living with dementia can face many challenges due to poor environmental design. Potential hazards and obstacles include a lack of suitable seating, a lack of wheelchair access and poorly maintained paths.

Another barrier was an assumption among some staff, and within the approach to everyday life taken by organizations, that going outdoors was risky for residents generally and people living with dementia in particular – for example, the possibility that someone might have a fall and hurt themselves. This could be addressed by taking a more person-centred approach based on a wide range of nature-based, positive risk-taking activities with people living with dementia and summarized by Mapes (2017) with the phrase 'Think Outside'. Mapes describes how positive risk-taking means supporting someone to get outside by finding out what people want to do, not letting fear cloud our judgement and minimizing risks through improving the environment, building confidence and allowing room for 'just being outdoors' (Mapes 2017: 164).

Other reasons given for not going outdoors included extreme weather and staff shortages. Most challenges to getting outside can be overcome with sufficient thought and planning, but when someone really cannot get outdoors or doesn't want to, there are plenty of ways to 'bring the outdoors in'. These include nature-based craft sessions, indoor gardening and visits from animals. For example, residents of one care home in the 'green care' study enjoyed regular indoor visits from guinea pigs and dogs from charitable organizations, while people moving into some extra care housing schemes had brought a cat with them. Several personal reasons were also given for limited access to the outdoors, the most common being reduced mobility due to illness and injury. One participant commented, 'When you have arthritis and you ache everywhere, it is not easy.'

A project focusing on supported housing found that enabling tenants to walk around both indoors and outside presented challenges for staff in terms of recognizing the benefits, knowing how to respond supportively and feeling too busy to do so (Barrett et al. 2020). This activity is referred to negatively as 'wandering', which obscures the fact that it is purposeful and meaningful, often motivated by historical events in someone's life including a desire to get outdoors. Common responses to spontaneous walking outdoors in domestic housing settings included keeping doors locked, something which raises serious issues of deprivation of liberty and infringes social citizenship. This study also concluded that a preferred name for this behaviour is 'walking with purpose'.

The natural environment, identity and citizenship

Some people living with dementia struggle with maintaining a sense of their own identity, possibly due to loss of memory about their own lives and interests (Caddell and Clare 2010) but also because of how they are treated by other people (Sabat and Harré 1992). Being outdoors and taking part in activities that someone has previously enjoyed, such as walking and gardening, can enable people living with dementia to reconnect with their past lives and boost a sense of identity. In the outdoor activity project mentioned earlier, a member of staff described how one participant, Keith, was painting a wall. During this activity he became covered in paint and at the end he said: 'I love that. I haven't done that for years, I felt like a man.'

One component of self-identity is a feeling of belonging to where we live, sometimes known as place attachment. Livingstone (1995) defined place attachment as the emotional bonds individuals have to particular places, including the neighbourhood in which they live. He suggested that we make stronger bonds with a place if it meets our physical and psychological needs and matches our goals and lifestyle. The longer we live in one place, the closer our sense of identity and self-esteem becomes entwined with our sense of belonging to places and our interactions with the people who we share those places with. Natural places that can be easily accessed and used by people living with dementia for a range of leisure activities, such as walking locally, can enhance feelings of belonging and community attachment for people living with dementia (Phinney et al. 2016).

Specific physical features in the environment can contribute towards a strong sense of identity with place (Munro 1995). These might be a natural landmark, such as a tree or a hill, or a particular building. A modern example of this approach can be seen in new urban developments such as the Millennium Village in Greenwich, London, where the grouping of houses around a green or lake are attempts to create social connections that focus on strong place-based features. Although social networks increasingly extend far beyond the immediate locality and often include online connections, communities focused on the local neighbourhood are still important, especially among older people and particularly those with family and friends close by (Nash and Christie 2003). The concept of 'civic memory' is also relevant here, whereby the history and features of a neighbourhood can contribute towards a sense of place and community as well as individual identity (Graham et al. 2009). Therefore, enabling opportunities to engage with the local natural environment and landscape through leisure activities can support the maintenance of memory, identity and well-being (Lengen and Kistemann 2012).

Having opportunities to take part in nature-based leisure activities such as gardening is also relevant to the concept of social citizenship, whereby people living with dementia have a right to active participation in their own lives and in society (Nedlund et al. 2019). This includes interaction with others, often a feature of nature-based activities such as walking. Similarly, nature-based activities emphasize the value of participation of people with dementia in leisure, which is a key aspect of their positioning as citizens with a valued role to play in wider society. Nedlund and colleagues recognized that being a 'good' citizen depends on many of the abilities that can be impaired because of dementia, such as communication, organization and reasoning. They suggest that access is a key element of inclusive citizenship, and that for people living with dementia this also includes the right to access resources, places and opportunities for connecting with nature.

Concluding thoughts

Connecting with nature through a range of leisure activities is highly valued and can bring a wealth of benefits in terms of health and well-being. However, many people living with dementia have reduced opportunities to enjoy nature, to experience 'the nourishing soil of the soul', often due to barriers to accessing outdoor spaces. This can have substantial negative impacts, including a loss of identity for those who have previously had a particular interest in outdoor activities such as walking and gardening. With all the benefits that experiencing nature can bring, ensuring safe access to nature for people living with dementia is therefore not only good practice, but also a matter of social citizenship, human rights and engagement with valued leisure activity.

So what does this mean in practice?

For those supporting or enabling the involvement in leisure of people living with dementia

- Having opportunities to connect with nature is important to the physical, social, emotional and spiritual well-being of people living with dementia.
- Anyone can be supported to connect with nature, but some creative and innovative thinking may be required.
- It is important to take a person-centred approach to connecting with nature, drawing on each individual's preferences and abilities.
- Easy access is key, and may require changes to the built environment.

For people living with dementia or their informal or family carers

- People living with dementia should insist on having opportunities to connect with nature if this is their wish.
- Those offering support should be advised of the person's interests and preferences in terms of nature.

For researchers

- The views of people living with dementia and their carers must be put at the heart of research into connecting with nature.

Endnote

1 Information and tools available from: https://www.worcester.ac.uk/about/academic-schools/school-of-allied-health-and-community/allied-health-research/association-for-dementia-studies/ads-consultancy/the-kings-fund-environmental-assessment-tools/

References

Barrett, J., Evans, S. and Mapes, N. (2019) Green dementia care in accommodation and care settings: A literature review, *Housing, Care and Support*, 22(4): 193–206.

Barrett, J., Evans, S. and Pritchard-Wilkes, V. (2020) Understanding and supporting safe walking with purpose among people living with dementia in extra care, retirement and domestic housing, *Housing, Care and Support*, 23(2): 37–48.

Buse, C. and Balmer, A. (2021) *My Home, My Garden Story: Exploring how People Living with Dementia Access and Use their Garden in Everyday Life*. York: University of York. Available at: http://www.york.ac.uk/media/sociology/52175_Dementia%20 and%20Gardens%20report-HR2-proof.pdf (accessed 2 March 2022).

Caddell, L.S. and Clare, L. (2010) The impact of dementia on self and identity: A systematic review, *Clinical Psychology Review*, 30(1): 113–26.

Evans, S.C., Barrett, J., Mapes, N. et al. (2019) Connections with nature for people living with dementia, *Working with Older People*, 23(3): 142–51.

Evans, S.C., Waller, S. and Bray, J. (2021) Designing inclusive environments for people living with dementia: How much do we really know?, *Working with Older People*, 26(2): 89–96.

Gonzalez, M.T. and Kirkevold, M. (2015) Clinical use of sensory gardens and outdoor environments in Norwegian nursing homes: A cross-sectional e-mail survey, *Issues in Mental Health Nursing*, 36(1): 35–43.

Graham, H., Mason, R. and Newman, A. (2009) *Literature Review: Historic Environment, Sense of Place, and Social Capital*. Newcastle: Newcastle University.

Hendriks, I.H., Vliet, D. van, Gerritsen, D.L. et al. (2016) Nature and dementia: Development of a person-centered approach, *International Psychogeriatrics*, 28(9): 1455–70.

Kaplan, S. (1995) The restorative benefits of nature: Toward an integrative framework, *Journal of Environmental Psychology*, 15(3): 169–82.

Lee, J., Park, B.-J., Tsunetsugu, Y. et al. (2011) Effect of forest bathing on physiological and psychological responses in young Japanese male subjects, *Public Health*, 125(2): 93–100.

Lengen, C. and Kistemann, T. (2012) Sense of place and place identity: Review of neuro-scientific evidence, *Health & Place*, 18(5): 1162–71.

Livingstone, D.N. (1995) The spaces of knowledge: Contributions towards a historical geography of science, *Environment and Planning D: Society and Space*, 13(1): 5–34.

Mapes, N. (2017) Think outside: Positive risk-taking with people living with dementia, *Working with Older People*, 21(3): 157–66.

Mensah, C.A., Andres, L., Perera, U. and Roji, A. (2016) Enhancing quality of life through the lens of green spaces: A systematic review approach, *International Journal of Well-being*, 6(1): 142–63.

Motealleh, P., Moyle, W., Jones, C. and Dupre, K. (2019) Creating a dementia-friendly environment through the use of outdoor natural landscape design intervention in long-term care facilities: A narrative review, *Health & Place*, 58: 102148.

Munro, G. (1995) Sense of place in towns, historic buildings as cultural icons, in J.M. Fladmark (ed.) *Sharing the Earth: Local Identity in Global Culture*. London: Donhead Publishing, pp. 325–31.

Nash, V. and Christie, I. (2003) *Making Sense of Community*. London: Institute for Public Policy Research.

Nedlund, A-C., Bartlett R. and Clarke, C. (2019) *Everyday Citizenship and People with Dementia*. Edinburgh: Dunedin.

Phinney, A., Kelson, E., Baumbusch, J. et al. (2016) Walking in the neighbourhood: Performing social citizenship in dementia, *Dementia*, 15(3): 381–94.

Sabat, S.R. and Harré, R. (1992) The construction and deconstruction of self in Alzheimer's Disease, *Ageing and Society*, 12(4): 443–61.

Spracklen, K. (2013) *Leisure, Sports and Society*. Basingstoke: Palgrave Macmillan.

Wilson, E.O. (1984) *Biophilia: The Human Bond with Other Species*. London: Harvard University Press.

12 Dementia access in museums and galleries

Nuala Morse, Zoe Brown, Sophie Mitchell, Joanne Charlton, Julianna Thompson and Helen Chatterjee

Summary

Museums and galleries are places for curiosity, creativity and learning. They often have distinctive architecture and display objects and stories with historical importance and personal significance. But they can also sometimes be difficult for people living with dementia to access. Physical adjustments and staff training can help make them welcoming and enabling places for people visiting independently or with others. In this chapter we look at guidance and examples of good practice for this in the UK and internationally, highlighting what is important and unique about museums as spaces of leisure. We then take a closer look at the programme at Tyne & Wear Archives & Museums (TWAM) in the UK, where the focus is on people's creative capabilities not their deficits. This programme also demonstrates how museums can provide opportunities for cultural engagement inside and outside of the museum. For example, activity loans boxes mean people engage with museum objects and creative activities in care homes and in hospitals. TWAM has also developed training and resources for health and social care professionals to use museum activities in their own practice. Examples like this show the importance of physical access and welcoming environments, and of celebrating everyone's creativity. They also show that dementia-friendly cultural leisure provision can be created both inside museums and in the community through outreach activities.

Considering museums and galleries as leisure spaces

Through their distinctive architectural venues and their collections of historical and personal significance, museums and galleries provide unique sites for leisure. Museums can be spaces of quiet contemplation and relaxation, or spaces of conviviality for family visits and through interactions with staff. Museums are places where people go to learn, but also to experience emotions and to have fun. They are associated with a sense of place, and of community, and with opportunities for supporting people to engage with issues of identity and of meaning. Previous studies have recognized 'museum visits' as part of meaningful leisure activities for people living with dementia (Yates et al. 2016). Intervention and observational studies relating to well-being programmes for people living with dementia and their carers delivered by museums, galleries and heritage sites have demonstrated a range of benefits including opportunities for intellectual engagement, social engagement, light physical activity, relaxation and enjoyment (e.g. Camic et al. 2014, 2016, 2017; Belver et al. 2018; Hendriks et al. 2021; Innes et al. 2021).

In the UK, US and Europe, some museums and galleries are part of a new movement by cultural organizations aiming to enable those living with dementia to benefit from their spaces and their collections. In the UK, where many of the examples discussed in this chapter are based, this has been driven by an accessibility (or access) agenda within legal frameworks and sector guidance (Smith et al. 2012). Much of this discourse is based on the social model of disability (Barnes 2019), which states that disability is caused by societal barriers that prevent or restrict people with impairments from fully taking part in community life. Following this model, the responsibility sits with museums and art galleries to ensure their buildings and programming are accessible to all (Dodd and Sandell 2001), and within this, to take forward specific considerations for including people living with dementia.

Many museums may not be immediately accessible for people living with dementia. Barriers to access may be physical as well as financial, attitudinal or cultural; it is well known that museums and galleries have a long history of elitism and exclusion. Previous studies using census data in both the UK and Europe have shown that adults with a long-standing illness or impairment are significantly less likely to visit museums or galleries, to the extent that across European contexts they are 12 percentage points more likely to have no visits at all (Falk and Katz-Gerro 2016). Research by Age UK (2018) identifies the main barriers to accessing creative and cultural activities (including museum visits) for older people as lack of transport, lack of support to get out and attend and lack of knowledge of what is available in the local area. While there has not been a comprehensive review of barriers for people living with dementia, it is likely that there are similar challenges to their fully enjoying museums and galleries as leisure spaces.

To address this in the UK the museum sector has been working in partnership with the Alzheimer's Society to improve access. Several English language dementia-friendly toolkits have been produced to provide specific accessibility guidance for cultural organizations (see Table 12.1 below). These are authored by museums or consortia (such as the UK's Age-Friendly Museum network) together with people living with dementia and support organizations. Each makes a clear case for becoming more dementia-friendly (here adapted from the 2015 *Dementia-Friendly Arts Guide*, see Table 12.1):

- There is a moral case, as everyone should have access to the arts and culture.
- There is a health and well-being case, linked to the growing evidence for the positive effects of arts and culture on the physical and mental health of people living with dementia.

- There is an artistic case, as working with and alongside people living with dementia can inspire artists' creativity.
- There is a strong business case, as people living with dementia represent a large and mostly untapped leisure audience.

This chapter begins with a review of the dementia-friendly toolkits available, which suggests that making venues dementia-friendly is about physical access, signage and wayfinding, but also much more: it is about how museums communicate their offer, about raising awareness among staff to create welcoming spaces and about working in partnership with support organizations and directly with people living with dementia to create opportunities for people to actively enjoy, participate in, shape and create culture. The movement for dementia-friendly museums can be conceived as supporting the movement for 'living well with dementia' by presenting museums as meaningful spaces of leisure.

We provide examples of dementia-friendly initiatives in museums and art galleries to consider the efforts across the sector in reconfiguring the museum as a space of leisure for people living with dementia. Our chapter also draws on published studies relating to several of these programmes to establish some of the distinctive features of museums as spaces for leisure. We then offer a detailed case study of the *Platinum Programme* from Tyne & Wear Archives & Museums (TWAM). We are writing as a group of researchers and museum practitioners who have collaborated on TWAM's dementia-friendly museum initiatives and evaluated their impact. TWAM is a local authority museum, art gallery and archive service with nine venues in the north-east of England and internationally significant collections in archives, art, science and technology, archaeology, military and social history, fashion and natural sciences. The *Platinum Programme* focuses on people aged 55 years and over with a range of additional health needs, and also provides tailored activity for people living with dementia. It includes supported independent visits, tailored programming and outreach activity in care homes and hospitals. At the heart of TWAM's approach is a commitment to working with people by putting lived experience at the heart of programming. While dominant approaches to ageing have been organized around illness and deficit, with dementia seen as loss (including of memory and physical function), the TWAM programme focuses on people's capabilities. The *Platinum Programme* is designed to enable people living with dementia to explore TWAM's collections, to connect directly with local culture and heritage and to create community groups and friendships. Across the programme, the focus is celebrating the creativity of every participant and recognizing their contribution to shaping culture and society more widely. In these ways, the example of TWAM shows how, when specific considerations are taken for welcoming people living with dementia, museums can play a valued role in supporting social citizenship.

The TWAM programme is also notable in providing a range of leisure activities both inside and outside of the museums, and in working in partnership to integrate cultural activities into formal care pathways. This further extends the locations within which people living with dementia can engage with leisure across community spaces, creating opportunities for cultural participation in a more democratic, unbounded manner. Drawing from the overview of practice and the case study of TWAM, we then summarize key learning on how museums and galleries can provide unique and stimulating environments to support the active creative and social lives of people living with dementia.

Museum and gallery initiatives for people living with dementia: an overview

To inform this chapter, six toolkits for museums and arts organization were identified in a rapid review conducted by the authors. These present numerous dementia-friendly initiatives and dedicated programming in museums and galleries of all kinds and sizes. The overview below primarily examines UK-based examples along with some international ones, focusing on the key areas identified in the review of dementia-friendly toolkits: accessibility, programming and partnerships. It also draws on published studies to help highlight some of the distinct features of museums seen as spaces of leisure. Details of the toolkits included can be found in Table 12.1, below.

Accessibility

Accessible environments are key to supporting those living with dementia and their partners to continue engaging with culture independently. The accessibility standards identified across the review of dementia-friendly guidance (Table 12.1) include the provision of physically accessible facilities, wayfinding and signage, adequate seating for rest and dedicated quiet spaces, as well as design consideration (e.g. avoiding patterns on floors that might be confusing, appearing as holes, steps or as wet surfaces) and appropriate and inclusive communication. At the Museum of London, for example, to help those with dementia navigate the galleries, visitors can access sensory maps of the museum that highlight quiet and loud areas. Across guidance it is also noted that creating accessible environments extends beyond the building itself to include acknowledgment of the wider context of the museum visit, including accessible websites with signposted travel options.

Another aspect of accessibility is ensuring that people living with dementia feel welcomed by staff. In the UK, there has been significant investment in staff training through partnership with the Alzheimer's Society's national Dementia Friends training programme. This raises awareness of the condition and its challenges to ensure staff are equipped to support visitors living with dementia. Such awareness can help to move accessibility issues beyond physical matters to wider environmental adjustments and behaviour change, ensuring museums and galleries are welcoming and supportive leisure spaces that people living with dementia can access independently with care partners. Staff training has been noted across studies as important for creating a sense of

Table 12.1 English-language dementia-friendly toolkits for museums and galleries

Toolkit	Authors	Publisher	Audience	Key contents	Museum and art gallery case studies
Dementia-Friendly Arts Guide: A Practical Guide to Becoming a Dementia-Friendly Arts Venue (2015)	A. Allen, A. Brown, P. Camic, D. Cutler, L. Harvey, M. Pasiecznik Parsons, R. Sweeney, E. Ward, H. Zeilig	Alzheimer's Society (UK)	Large and small arts venues, art galleries and museums	• Key information on dementia • Raising awareness in organizations • Programming and processes • Facilities • Further resources • Appendix: research and evaluation in the arts and dementia care	Dulwich Picture Gallery Historic Royal Palaces Manchester Museum and Whitworth Art Gallery National Museums Liverpool
Handbook for cultural engagement with people living with dementia		The Whitworth (UK)	Museums and art galleries	• Key information about dementia • Top tips from people living with dementia • Lessons learned • Visitor feedback • Impact	
Age-Friendly Museum Toolkit (2019)		Museum Development North West (UK)	Small and large museums and art galleries	• Age-friendly standards • Building relationships • Programming • Facilities • Communication • Providing a warm welcome	Victoria Gallery & Museum, Liverpool Merseyside Fire and Rescue Service Heritage and Education Centre Haworth Art Gallery National Football Museum Towneley Hall Art Gallery & Museum

(continued)

Table 12.1 *(continued)*

Toolkit	Authors	Publisher	Audience	Key contents	Museum and art gallery case studies
Dementia Toolkit		Tunbridge Wells Museum and Art Gallery (UK)	Small to medium museums	• How to develop object-handling sessions for people living with dementia • How a session works and why • Evaluation	
Rethinking Heritage: A Guide To Help Make Your Site More Dementia-Friendly (2017)	K. Klug, S. Page, J. Connell, D. Robson, E. Bould	Historic Royal Palaces (UK)	Heritage sites	• Key information about dementia • How dementia can affect a heritage visit • Visitor experience • Partnership • Programming • Common challenges for the heritage sector	
Health and Wellbeing in Museums Toolkit (2021)		The Beaney House of Art and Knowledge (UK)	Small and large museums	• Understanding health and well-being (including dementia) • Recruitment • Planning activities • Measuring impact • Funding	Tunbridge Wells Museum and Art Gallery

support and safety for people living with dementia during museum visits (Roe et al. 2016).

Several UK museums now have a clear statement on their website about their commitment to being a dementia-friendly organization. The Manchester Museum, the Whitworth Art Gallery and Beamish – The Living Museum of the North have trained all their visitor-facing staff (learning, volunteers and visitor teams) to become Dementia Friends. In 2019, The National Trust committed to make all five hundred historic and countryside homes dementia-friendly, and to a review of policies and processes to support volunteers who may be affected by dementia. At the Museum of London, staff training extends to the museum Directorate, to ensure all levels of the institution are committed to dementia access. In 2021, the Mayor of London and the Alzheimer's Society launched the world's first *Dementia-Friendly Venues Charter*, which includes a Dementia-Friendly Arts and Culture Network delivered by the Museum of London, with 40 signatories across major cultural venues in the UK capital. With clear toolkits, training and charters available, there is scope for museums to continue to develop their accessibility standards for people living with dementia.

Programming

As stated in the *Dementia-Friendly Arts Guide* (Allen et al. 2015: 18), dementia-friendly programming is about 'presenting things in ways that enable visitors with dementia – and their carers – to relax, engage with and enjoy the experience'. This is a useful definition for understanding the potential of museums as leisure spaces. There are several examples of dedicated creative programmes for people living with dementia and their partners, including supported visits and tours, arts-based and sensory activities, cafes and social events. A founding initiative is the *Meet Me at MoMA* programme from the Museum of Modern Art in New York. Since 2007, MoMA has been delivering in-gallery discussion for people living with dementia and their care partners (Rosenberg 2009). These are small group tours of selected art works and a group discussion facilitated by specially trained museum educators. MoMA has developed extensive resources for other museums to replicate this approach, freely available on their website. This has inspired practice across the world – for instance, the *Unforgettable* programme at the Van Abbemuseum in Amsterdam (Hendriks et al. 2021). *Coffee, Cake and Culture* at the Whitworth Art Gallery in Manchester is another example of a free, two-hour guided visit fully supported by artists and volunteers (Roe et al 2016).

Museum programming also includes arts-based and sensory group activities, with examples of practice found internationally across different types of art galleries and museums in Italy, France, Lithuania, Germany, the Netherlands, Australia and the USA. These range from art-making sessions and memory cafes using collections, to meditation and movement activities. For example, the Museum of London delivers the *Memories of London* programme, with a number of strands, including self-led creative activity packs; *London Lives*, a podcast series featuring the voices and stories of people living with dementia; and the monthly *Time for a Cuppa* sessions, with museum objects, stories and songs in the gallery. Historic Royal Palaces runs *Sensory Palaces*, a multisensory storytelling exploration of its heritage sites (Innes et al. 2021). Most of these programmes are free for people living with dementia and their care partners, with programmes funded through a mixture of external and core funding.

Ensuring the activities are meaningful, engaging and enjoyable to participants lies at the heart of successful programming. Research studies have examined the well-being impact of dementia-friendly programming, including viewing art in a gallery setting, on people living with dementia and their care partners. These highlight (albeit briefly) some of the unique features of programmes set in museum spaces. Participants noted the significance of museums as 'valued', 'trusted', 'special' and 'prestigious' settings linked to their architecture or their historical importance. Accessing such spaces made people feel privileged and important, as well as offering important distraction from everyday worries (Camic et al. 2014, 2016). Most significantly, inclusion in activity in cultural spaces enabled participants to feel themselves to be active and valued members of society. This gives some further insight into the distinctive nature of museums and the potential importance of culture in enjoying full lives for people living with dementia.

Partnerships

At the heart of the types of programming discussed above are partnerships with charities and support organizations for people living with dementia. Partnership is identified as key to the success of programmes across various toolkits, which often cite the importance of learning directly from those with lived experience of dementia and their care partners. One significant partnership is the *House of Memories* programme at National Museums Liverpool; this offers training, resources and museum-based activities to support carers for people living with dementia with practical skills and confidence to visit museums.

Another type of partnership work in museums is focused on co-producing exhibitions that address lived experience of dementia. In 2018, The Whitworth Art Gallery in Manchester presented *Beyond Dementia*, an exhibition exploring how to live well with a diagnosis of dementia. The exhibition was curated by the Fabulous Forgetful Friends, a local group invited by the museum to select artworks from the collection for display, presented alongside their own art, personal stories and text panels challenging negative perceptions of dementia. The public message of the exhibition was to encourage visitors to see the person beyond the illness and diagnosis. The Fabulous Forgetful Friends also contributed to an accompanying publication, *A Handbook for Cultural Engagement with People Living with Dementia* (2018), where they ask that museum professionals engage them with 'respect, dignity and humour', reminding professionals not to underestimate what they are capable of. While there are currently only a few examples like this from practice, involving people living with dementia to tell their stories in museum spaces can play an important role in supporting active social citizenship by giving voice to people's experiences and by challenging societal stigma.

Tyne & Wear Archives & Museums *Platinum Programme:* extending leisure opportunities for wider inclusion

The *Platinum Programme* at TWAM was launched in 2014 as an overarching programme of activity for older adults (over 55) and people living with dementia, led by the Outreach Team as part of their *Adult Health and Well-being Programme.* The programme aims to provide meaningful activities both inside and outside of museums, to encourage social interaction and develop the creative capabilities of those living with dementia and those caring for them. The *Platinum Programme* adopts a positive perspective on ageing and active citizenship, going beyond reminiscence work only[1] to focus on inspiration, imagination and learning, with an emphasis on person-centred care (Kitwood 1997). This is significant when thinking about programmes through the lens of social citizenship (or a quality of life paradigm) in recognition of the range of creative capabilities held by people living with dementia and moving beyond the focus on memory loss. The programme has varied strands of activity that provide opportunities for people with different needs, for those living independently and those in care homes or hospitals, and specialized training opportunities for health and social care staff to access creative professional development. Every strand uses the wide variety of TWAM collections and venues to offer dementia-friendly activities. The programme is delivered by trained museum professionals, with a focus on creating accessible, safe and friendly environments for enjoyable leisure. Each strand provides a bespoke offer to enable wider inclusion of people living with dementia.

Slow Museums

Slow Museums aims to encourage those who feel isolated, anxious or who lack confidence to come into the museum venues, in particular those living with dementia. The monthly afternoons are based on the model of 'slow shopping',[2] and aim to provide an enabling environment to anyone who needs it. Practical arrangements include providing extra seating in galleries, turning down a particularly loud exhibition or turning lighting up if needed (just for a few hours, as bright lights can damage museum displays). The museum provides extra clear signage and maps to aid navigation, and museum handling objects for visitors to touch and interact with. Cafe and administration staff have also had extra training, so they are aware of visitors' needs during that afternoon. *Slow Museums* opens up and adjusts the space of the museum for successful independent visiting.

Coffee, Cake and Culture

Coffee, Cake and Culture is a supported programme that provides a range of activity in venues, such as behind-the-scenes tours, meetings with curators, object handling sessions and inspiring conversation – always over tea and cake. Activities respond to current and temporary exhibitions to offer a changing programme of supported leisure activities for older adults that is inclusive of people living with dementia and their care partners. A key focus of the activities is a relaxed environment facilitated by staff for participants to engage with a variety of themes and collections at their own pace. *Coffee, Cake and Culture* is an example of enabling people living with dementia to access all areas in the museums through dedicated supported activity.

Time Travellers

In 2015, Age UK North Tyneside approached TWAM about including Segedunum Roman Fort in their plans to make Wallsend town centre dementia-friendly. To support these plans, the museum set up a weekly programme of activities for people living with dementia and their care partners, which participants chose to call *Time Travellers*. Weekly activities were based on different time periods using museum handling objects, from prehistory, to Roman and Egyptian times, to the 1950s and 1970s. Over time, participants took ownership of the programme, devising themes for weekly meetings and bringing in their own photographs and objects to share their stories. As an outcome of *Time Travellers*, group members reported that they had made new friends, had increased self-esteem from being listened to and felt their sense of self reaffirmed by sharing their own memories. Carers also reported positive outcomes from attending

Figure 12.1 Time Travellers Audrey and Christine at Segedunum Roman Fort, Tyne & Wear Archives & Museums

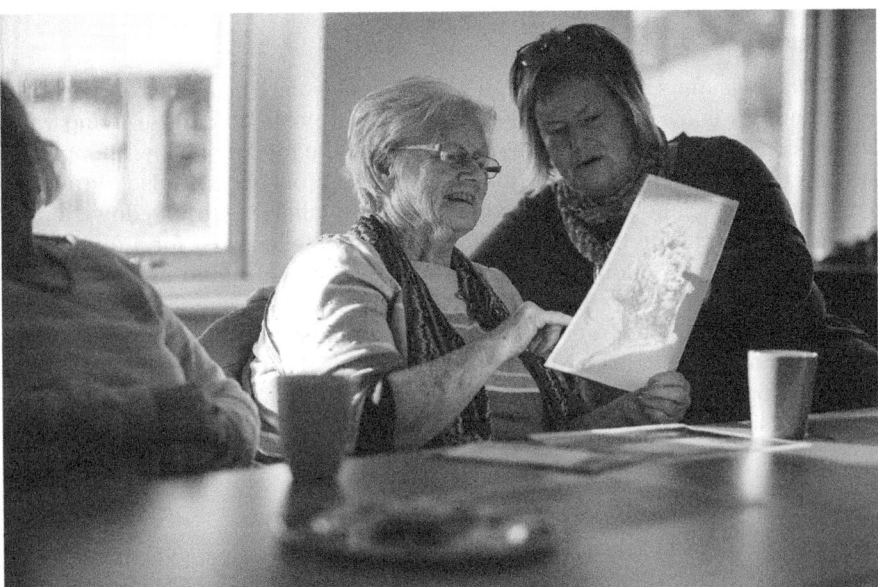

the group. *Time Travellers* is an example where the museum acts as a local space that fosters social citizenship and community, and where people living with dementia shape their own cultural leisure activities.

Activity loans boxes and outreach

Handling boxes have been developed by the museum team with objects that are taken out to different groups, care homes, lunch clubs and local history groups. These contain a range of everyday original objects primarily from the 1940s and 1950s, memorabilia, newspapers, photographs, sounds recordings and clothing. The boxes have a range of different themes, including Childhood, Entertainment, Fashion, Holidays, Shopping, Home Life and Work Life. They can be used to bring back memories and to create fun, with tactile activities that spark discussion. The aim is not to act only as memory boxes but rather to enable open-ended exploration of materials and artefacts from the past. Boxes are used by museum professionals to support outreach sessions, and they can also be borrowed directly by care homes. Each box comes with resources and ideas for creative activities so that care home staff can use the boxes independently. The boxes enable the museum to travel into other places, supporting cultural engagement for those who may not be able to visit, therefore extending leisure opportunities through outreach activity.

Figure 12.2 A childhood-themed museum activity loans box

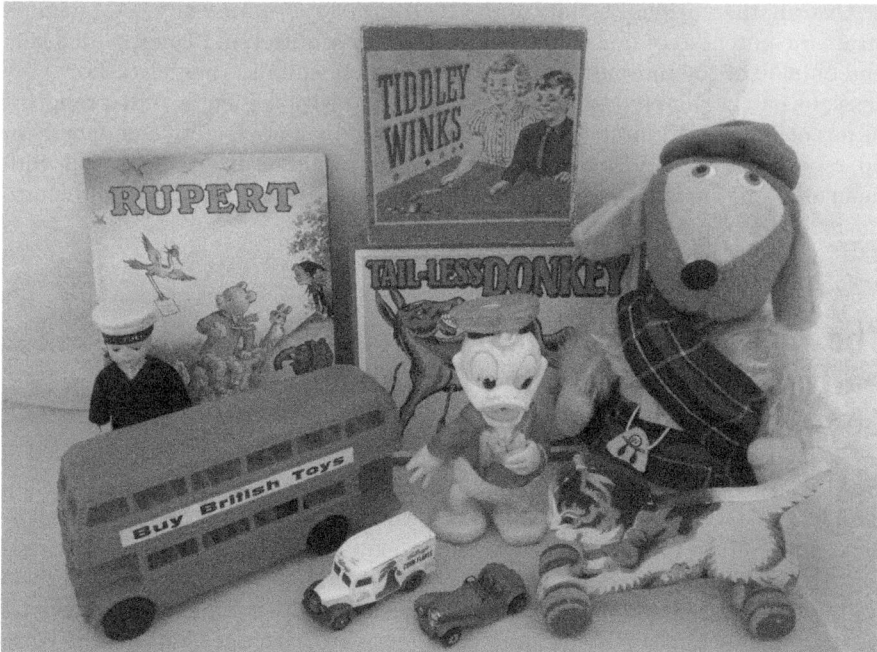

Between 2015 and 2018, TWAM was involved in a research project with University College London, funded by Arts Council England, to investigate the health and well-being benefits of museum-based engagement (Not So Grim Up North Research Team 2018). As part of the research, TWAM developed a series of workshops with the Castleside inpatient dementia services ward at The Centre for Ageing and Vitality in Newcastle upon Tyne. This is a secure unit for people with severe dementia, so sessions were adapted to meet more complex needs and the requirements of a formal care setting, thinking of the content, slower pace and increased facilitator ratio. The museum sessions were centred on using objects from the 1940s and took place weekly over two hours, supported by a museum worker and ward staff, with a focus on sensory engagement and conversation for in-the-moment enjoyment and relaxation. A small intervention study observed seven people (four of them male) and found that, for many participants observed, positive emotions increased over the time of the sessions (Morse et al. 2020). The study also examined social interaction, and there were suggestions that the activity provided opportunities for positive engagement between staff and patients. What appeared key to the success of these sessions was the patience, compassion and level of attention from the museum worker that enabled everyone to participate as much as they felt able over the length of the session, often in short bursts, but sometimes over a more sustained period. The project also allowed care staff to engage in a fun activity with patients and to get to know people differently. This research shows that museum activities can be a positive meaningful leisure activity in the context of severe dementia care in hospital settings.

Overall, the various strands of the *Platinum Programme* at TWAM demonstrate the potential of museum engagement across different places, both inside and outside of the museum, in care homes and hospitals. They also show how sessions can be adapted to include people living with dementia with a range of different needs and circumstances. Each strand supports active engagement by recognizing and celebrating the creative abilities of people living with dementia and providing the support needed in each case, welcoming them to the museum or meeting them where they are.

The Museum Health and Social Care Service: partnership and training for those who support people living with dementia

One key aspect of the innovative practice at TWAM is the focus on partnership with health and social care (H&SC) professionals to scale up opportunities for access to culture for those living with dementia. Like many museums, TWAM experienced limited staff capacity to deliver workshops, while the H&SC sectors had limited capability in terms of confidence and competency to develop heritage-themed activities as part of their care practices. In 2019, TWAM worked with Northumbria University Faculty for Health and Life Sciences to develop the *Museum, Health and Social Care Service* resource (MHSCS).[3] The MHSCS provides resources for H&SC professionals to build confidence and understanding of how to use museum resources in the care of older people, including people living with dementia. The resource is based on clinical frameworks of reference (the Comprehensive Geriatric Assessment) and presents the ways in which museum activities might support all domains of health and well-being – psychological and cognitive, social, functional, physical and environmental. Current research evidence suggests that many H&SC professionals rely primarily on clinical frameworks of reference to direct their care and struggle to regard art and heritage activities as relevant to their care delivery (Broome et al. 2017). One solution to this is to provide guidance about care and clinical benefits – i.e. bring these activities within the clinical frames of reference familiar to these professionals.

The resource was developed through a multidisciplinary collaboration consisting of museum outreach staff from TWAM, H&SC practitioners and academics (occupational therapists, physiotherapists, mental health nurses, social workers and older people's nurses), and older people using services. This ensured that all stakeholders were involved in the development, especially older adults and people living with dementia who would benefit directly. The MHSCS resource is unique in that it is searchable via required care outcomes. It then suggests appropriate activities and identifies how these could support the selected health/well-being outcomes – for example, pain management, mobility, nutrition/hydration, speech, cognitive stimulation, mental health or social interaction. The resource brings together the languages of both the arts, cultural and heritage world, and the H&SC context, promoting mutual understanding of the positive impact that arts, culture and heritage can have on health and well-being. Ultimately, the purpose of the resource is to support quality of life improvements for older people – as such it centres on providing meaningful and enjoyable activity that people can engage in freely and promotes creative agency alongside therapeutic and physical benefits.

The MHSCS has been rolled out across the north-east of England and is free to use. Alongside the resource, TWAM have developed training sessions and short instructive films that H&SC professionals can access to support their own facilitated heritage-themed workshops. Once trained, H&SC professionals can use 'activity loans boxes' provided by TWAM and containing materials required to do the MHSCS activities. The MHSCS is also part of the nursing curricula at Northumbria University, so that the future H&SC workforce will be confident and competent to apply arts, culture and heritage in their care practices from the point of professional registration.

Expanding the role for museums as spaces of leisure for people living with dementia

Museums play a key storytelling role in society. Exhibitions can be used to showcase the creative and artistic capacities of those living with dementia. Co-curation approaches can be an important means of empowering people living with dementia to find their voice and tell their stories on their own terms. There are perhaps fewer examples of practice in this area. Nonetheless, because museums are highly trusted institutions, they can play an important role in shaping societal discussions around mental health and living well in older age. There is further potential in using museums in presenting diverse experiences to reframe the stigmatizing discourse around dementia.

The range of evidence about the importance of cultural, art and heritage activities to the health and well-being of people living with dementia, combined with the rich wealth of practice examples and sector guidance we presented in this chapter, should act as a call for museums and art galleries to continue developing their provision. There is great potential here, given that museums provide opportunities for multisensory stimulation, which has also been recognized as useful in the treatment of dementia (Cheng et al. 2019). It is important to note, however, that there remain several gaps in understanding. Although the toolkits do provide best practice guidance, there is little overall research about the specific barriers faced by people living with dementia in accessing cultural provision. Additionally, very little research relates to the experiences of Black, Asian and other minority ethnic individuals with dementia in accessing cultural provision and the additional barriers they face. There is also much wider scope for research to investigate the specific features of museums and heritage that create unique and distinctive leisure spaces. These characteristics can be inferred from the literature we have reviewed here, but this has so far not been the specific focus of research which could yield a deeper understanding of the importance of culture within social citizenship for people living with dementia.

So what does this mean in practice?

For those supporting or enabling the involvement in leisure of people living with dementia

- The review of published toolkits makes clear that including people living with dementia is about both physical access – for example, seating, wayfinding and websites – *and* creating a welcoming, relaxed, safe and enjoyable environment for visitors.

- Staff training plays an important role here, as do partnerships with support organizations and directly with people living with dementia and their care partners to consult on access and provision. This helps to raise awareness about the condition, challenge stereotypes and ensure people are treated as active and valued members of society.

- The success of the programming relies on intent and delivery: no matter where or who is delivering the activity, it must centre people's creative capabilities and agency, focus on enjoyment and be supported by a welcoming, inclusive and positive attitude.

For people living with dementia or their informal or family carers

- Museums and galleries offer a range of leisure provision, from independent visits to supported group activities, as well as activities in community and care settings.

For researchers

- There is good evidence about the importance of cultural, art and heritage activities to the health and well-being of people living with dementia. There is scope for research to continue to investigate the *specific* features of museums and galleries that create unique and distinctive leisure spaces.
- Further research should continue to address the facilitators and barriers to access to account for diversity within experiences of dementia.

Endnotes

1   This has been noted as an early focus of many museum programmes for people living with dementia.
2   In the UK, the Slow Shopping social movement was founded by Katherine Vero in 2015 with the objective of providing a safe and welcoming environment for anyone needing to take more time to do their shopping. This YouTube video explains the concept: https://www.youtube.com/watch?v=4BZtgP2YPYk
3   The resource is available at https://www.twmuseums.org.uk/museums-health-and-social-care-service

References

Age UK (2018) *Creative and Cultural Activities and Wellbeing in Later Life.* Available at: https://www.ageuk.org.uk/creative-wellbeing/ (accessed 13 July 2022).

Allen, A., Brown, A., Camic, P. et al. (2015) *Dementia-Friendly Arts Guide: A Practical Guide to Becoming a Dementia-Friendly Arts Venue.* London: Alzheimer's Society.

Barnes, C. (2019) Understanding the social model of disability: Past, present and future, in N. Watson and S. Vehmas (eds) *Routledge Handbook of Disability Studies,* 2nd edn (pp. 441–57). London: Routledge.

Belver, M.H., Ullán, A.M., Avila, N. et al. (2018) Art museums as a source of well-being for people with dementia: An experience in the Prado Museum, *Arts & Health,* 10(3): 213–26.

Broome, E., Dening, T., Schneider, J. and Brooker, D. (2017) Care staff and the creative arts: Exploring the context of involving care personnel in arts interventions, *International Psychogeriatrics,* 29(12): 1979–91.

Camic, P.M., Baker, E.L. and Tischler, V. (2016) Theorizing how art gallery interventions impact people with dementia and their caregivers, *The Gerontologist,* 56(6): 1033–41.

Camic, P.M., Hulbert, S. and Kimmel, J. (2017) Museum object handling: A health-promoting community-based activity for dementia care, *Journal of Health Psychology*, 24(6): 787–98.

Camic, P.M., Tischler, V. and Pearman, C.H. (2014) Viewing and making art together: A multi-session art-gallery-based intervention for people with dementia and their carers, *Aging & Mental Health*, 18(2): 161–8.

Cheng, C., Baker G.B. and Dursun, S.M. (2019) Use of multisensory stimulation interventions in the treatment of major neurocognitive disorders, *Psychiatry and Clinical Psychopharmacology*, 29(4): 916–21.

Dodd, J. and Sandell, R. (2001) *Including Museums: Perspectives on Museums, Galleries and Social Inclusion*. Leicester: Research Centre for Museums and Galleries, University of Leicester.

Falk, M. and Katz-Gerro, T. (2016) Cultural participation in Europe: Can we identify common determinants?, *Journal of Cultural Economics*, 40(2): 127–62.

Hendriks, I., Meiland, F.J., Gerritsen, D.L. and Dröes, R.M. (2021) Evaluation of the 'Unforgettable' art programme by people with dementia and their care-givers, *Ageing & Society*, 41(2): 294–312.

Innes, A., Scholar, H.F., Haragalova, J. and Sharma, M. (2021) 'You come because it is an interesting place': The impact of attending a heritage programme on the well-being of people living with dementia and their care partners, *Dementia*, 20(6): 2133–51.

Kitwood, T.M. (1997) *Dementia Reconsidered: The Person Comes First*. Buckingham: Open University Press.

Morse, N., Thomson, L. and Chatterjee, H. (2020) The role of co-production methods in developing an observational tool for museums in health research for people living with dementia, *Sage Research Methods Cases: Medicine and Health*, January: 1–13. DOI: https://doi.org/10.4135/9781529710632.

Not So Grim Up North Research Team (2018) *Not So Grim Up North: Investigating the Health and Wellbeing Impacts of Museum and Gallery Activities for People living with Dementia, Stroke Survivors, and Mental Health Service-Users*. Available at: https://www.ucl.ac.uk/biosciences/sites/biosciences/files/2018-not-so-grim-up-north.pdf (accessed 13 July 2022).

Roe, B., McCormick, S., Lucas, T. et al. (2016) Coffee, cake & culture: Evaluation of an art for health programme for older people in the community, *Dementia*, 15(4): 539–59.

Rosenberg, F. (2009) The MoMA Alzheimer's Project: Programming and resources for making art accessible to people with Alzheimer's disease and their caregivers, *Arts & Health*, 1(1): 93–7.

Smith, H.L.J., Ginley, B. and Goodwin, H. (2012) Beyond compliance? Museums, disability and the law, in R. Sandell and E. Nightingale (eds) *Museums, Equality, and Social Justice* (pp. 83–95). London: Routledge.

Yates, L.A., Ziser, S., Spector, A. and Orrell, M. (2016) Cognitive leisure activities and future risk of cognitive impairment and dementia: Systematic review and meta-analysis, *International Psychogeriatrics*, 28(11): 1791–1806.

13 Walking football

Rhoda Macrae, Liz Carlin and Eilidh Macrae

Summary

Sports can be modified so that they are more accessible for certain groups of people. One example of this is walking football, which is a non-contact form of the game, played at a slower pace. Walking football is popular, and some walking football sessions have been designed and delivered for people living with dementia. In this chapter we investigate the experiences of people who were involved in a dementia-friendly walking football programme held in Hampden Park, Glasgow, Scotland. These walking football sessions were designed to provide participants with the chance to play walking football with others in a dementia-friendly environment. For example, the location was served by accessible transport links, and staff were on hand to support with extra wayfinding signage or escorting where needed. The sessions also provided opportunity for participants, along with their carers and supporters, to socialize before and after every set of games. Carers and supporters were offered a space to stay and watch the walking football sessions, or they could take time to themselves. To investigate the impact of theses sessions on those involved, interviews were carried out with the participants, their carers and supporters, and those who designed and ran the sessions. Good practice included ensuring the location was geographically accessible with local transport links and having staff on hand to support with directions. It involved helping participants, families and supporters before and after each session, as well as providing choice for carers on how they might use their time during the session. It also included using football artefacts to support people living with dementia understand the purpose of participation and where the sessions were taking place. The research showed that Hampden Park provided a unique setting that stimulated football memories among participants.

An overview of sport and dementia, modified sports and walking football

This chapter will explore the experiences of people who were involved in a dementia-friendly walking football (soccer) programme held in Hampden Park, Glasgow, Scotland. We observed and interviewed participants, their carers and supporters, and facilitators of this walking football programme. To inform best practice for similar programmes, we wanted to learn about the programme's impact on participants, and which aspects of its setting and structure were vital to its success.

Hampden Park, Scotland's national football stadium, is an impressive venue; it is familiar, culturally significant and a source of pride for many Scots. Most walking football sessions which are offered in community settings do not have the memories and cultural significance associated with Hampden. While our exploration focuses on the social impact on participants and the 'Hampden effect', we were also mindful to gather details on aspects of the sessions which were enhanced by the space, but which might still be replicable in other leisure settings providing walking football, and we offer these as recommendations later. We start our chapter with some context on sport and dementia, modified sports, and an introduction to walking football.

Within research focusing on ageing, sport is often noted as a positive form of leisure (Jenkin et al. 2016), with social participation in particular showing benefits for overall health in older adults (Sirven and Debrand 2008). In their review of sport participation for older adults, Jenkin et al. (2016) found health to be both a positive outcome of engagement but also a limitation to participation. With barriers to taking part for older adults often linked to reduced mobility or fear of injury, modified sports have become a popular way to encourage inclusive involvement (Jenkin et al. 2018).

Modified sports were established to promote alternative options for young people to participate in adult sports (Eime et al. 2015). These modifications were then extended to people with disabilities. Research by Kiuppis in 2018 highlighted, however, that even though activities might be adapted there often remains a lack of available transport to enable people to access the sporting venue. Many venues themselves remain inaccessible. Both factors promote a reliance on others for support, and we return to these matters later in the chapter.

Walking sports are a type of modified sports aimed at helping people to get into sport or to maintain an active lifestyle in later stages of life. They often focus on encouraging people over 50 to return to sport if there has been a gap in their participation, and they also offer a chance to meet and connect with new people. Developed in the UK in 2011, walking football was the first example of this (Jenkin et al. 2018), and other sports have followed – for example, walking basketball, rugby, cricket and netball. The popularity of walking football in the UK is clear, especially among men over 50 years of age, with dedicated organizations now established to support local groups and clubs to develop, recruit members and link with a network of other walking football groups. Walking football follows the basic premise and rules of football. The key differences are that participants are not allowed to run or slide tackle, and they need to have one foot in contact with the ground at all times (Football Association 2018). There has been only limited research into the impact of walking football on physical health and well-being. Focusing more on the social impact of participation, McEwan et al. (2019) found that weekly walking football sessions fostered social connections for participants. A key reason why participants became involved in the programme that was the subject of their study was that there was a link to a professional football club and stadium.

In the last decade there has been an increase in sports-based interventions for people living with dementia (Watchman and Tolson 2015; Watson et al. 2018). Studies have also examined the effect of physical activity on cognitive, physical and social functioning, on well-being, and on quality of life in people living with dementia. There are mixed findings. For example, Lamb et al. (2018) reported no slowing of cognitive impairment in people with mild to moderate dementia who engaged with exercise training programmes. Other studies found exercise for people with dementia did not impact on psychological or behavioural symptoms but did improve activities of daily living skills and physical and cognitive functions (McDermott et al. 2019).

The positive social connection effects of participation are clear, however. Motivators for involvement in preferred leisure activities include feeling socially connected through being together with other people, maintaining physical and emotional well-being and a positive sense of self (van Alphen et al. 2016; Farina et al. 2020). Russell (2020) found that, through physical activity and sport, people living with dementia were more able to shape an aspirational sense of their own identity and future, especially as these were often activities which could be inclusive of others they were close to, such as family carers.

A study into the impact of football participation on men with young onset dementia found the players experienced positive anticipation and enjoyment (Carone et al. 2016). It described 'the Notts County effect', the success of the session being related to the strong brand of the club, and a person-centred service in a 'dementia-free' environment (i.e. while people were together dementia was not a topic prioritized for discussion, and it was not a focus of the occasion). Therefore, when aiming to increase physical activity and sport participation for people living with dementia, research suggests that it may help to focus programmes on sports like football, which have strong cultural and often personal associations. Our research aimed to explore the social impact of dementia-friendly walking football on participants and their supporters, as well as the influence of the programme design and setting, namely Hampden Park.

The dementia-friendly walking football programme

A link worker employed by the charity Alzheimer Scotland, who was a passionate footballer, was tasked with exploring activity options for men living with dementia. While individuals were keen to play football, they found general walking football programmes inaccessible due to their support needs. In response, the link worker organized a pilot dementia-friendly walking football programme that ran for six months during 2019 at Hampden Park. Hampden Park, and the Scottish Football Museum based there, have long supported people living with dementia. For example, the museum hosts Football Memories Scotland, where football images and reminiscence activities can be accessed online.

Fourteen men from the local area were recruited and participated in this dementia-friendly walking football programme once a month on a Thursday afternoon, to coincide with the Thursday morning Football Memories Scotland programme. Volunteers and some participants from the morning reminiscence programme stayed on in the afternoon for the walking football.

Figure 13.1 Dementia-friendly walking football at Hampden Park. Players and volunteers celebrate!

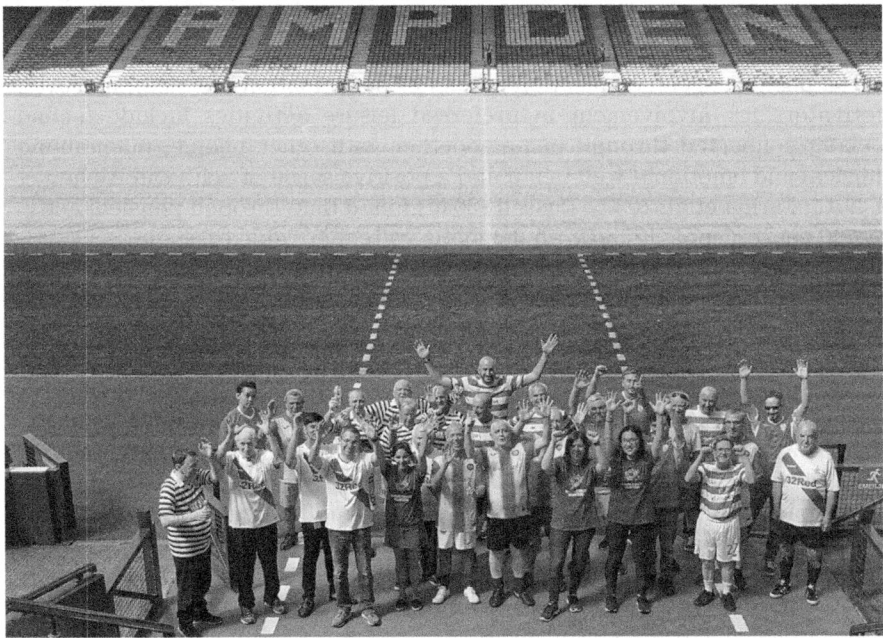

Before each session there was a good amount of person-centred support, with Alzheimer Scotland staff phoning participants and their supporters (family carers or paid carers) to go over directions, transport, options and the schedule. The afternoon programme lasted around two hours and began in the Hampden Cafe. The cafe is large and filled with football photographs and memorabilia. The volunteers then supported participants to go from the cafe to the changing rooms. In this space, participants were given the choice of a team strip from those donated by teams that play in the Glasgow Cup (Celtic, Rangers, Queens Park, Partick Thistle, Clyde and Third Lanark).

Each session took place in a small, indoor warm-up pitch situated between the changing rooms and the main stadium. They began with a short warm-up followed by 60 minutes of play, made up of ten-minute games. It was key that this play was flexible, and that the volunteers and staff were mindful of how participants were doing and allowed for breaks as required. Midway through, a longer break was taken. The purpose of this was twofold. It enabled a physical rest and an opportunity to walk out into the stadium through the main tunnel. There everyone could get some air, as well as pose for and take photographs. Being in the stadium reminded participants they were playing in the National Football Stadium, and the cultural relevance and personal meaning of this place for their identity and sense of self as football players and fans. After the break, the session resumed, and, at the end, after changing, participants left the Park.

Following the final session, information was provided for participants on options for continuing their involvement, such as walking football sessions in the wider area and Alzheimer Scotland's other community activities. There was also a post-programme celebration event in the Scottish Football Hall of Fame. For this, there was a museum tour, a prize-giving ceremony, and organizers had arranged for a former Glasgow Rangers and England international football player to speak.

The research participants

This study aimed to explore the social impact of dementia-friendly walking football to produce evidence that could inform its development. The research team worked with Alzheimer Scotland staff who were leading the existing walking football programme to invite participants and carers to take part in the research. To be included in the study the person had to be a participant, supporter or facilitator of the programme. Potential participants were provided with verbal and written information about the study with clear wording describing the research in a large font. The researcher used 'process consent,' checking in with participants during and between interviews to ensure they wished to continue participating, and primary carers were present during the interviews of any participants whose verbal ability was less strong.

Data collection: interviews and observations at Hampden Park

There were nine semi-structured interviews (in other words, interviews with some planned questions, but with flexibility to include additional questions if necessary) with participants, four with family carers, two with paid carers and two with programme staff. Contacts at the end of the programme comprised two interviews with players, two with family members and one with programme staff. Not as many players were able to take part in the later interviews due to deteriorated health, and because this was conducted at Christmas, a busy time, when an interview would have further disrupted routine.

The participants who were players (all men over 70) resided in different settings: five lived in a care home, and four lived at home with a family member acting as primary carer, such as a wife or daughter. Their dementia had progressed to varying degrees; all participants had memory, communication and language impairment, and for a few this disrupted their speech.

Initial interviews with participants who lived in their own homes took place at Hampden Park. For those who lived in a care home the interview took place in the entertainment room of the care home, which was recently used to watch a football match, and activity coordinators were present at these interviews. It was important that these spaces provided environmental prompts to frame the context and encourage familiarity for participants.

Questions asked during the interviews with the players focused on gaining an understanding of their mood, energy, social interactions and general health and well-being. This included exploring their footballing background if any, how they felt playing football again, and what they liked about the sessions as well as what they would change. The interviews with carers focused on how they felt the sessions had impacted on the men in relation to the same key areas of mood, social interactions and health and well-being. In addition, interviews with programme staff and volunteers explored their views of whether the programme required any adjustments to ensure it met the needs of participants.

Data were also gathered through observations, including all aspects from arrival, and the journey through Hampden Park to the cafe, changing room and pitch. This allowed researchers to see the social gatherings before and after sessions, the physical warm-ups and the sessions themselves, for both participants and the spectators. Observations focused on the frequency and type of interactions the men had with family members, carers, staff and other participants, as well as interactions between family members. Body language, observable mood and nature of participation during the sessions also formed key elements of this observational data.

The following section presents the findings from the observational and interview data under subheadings that draw out the importance of different spaces within Hampden Park.

The 'Hampden effect'

Participants used several different spaces within Hampden Park. This section frames findings based on how spaces were used by participants as they engaged with the sessions. Additionally, the place itself was important in enhancing the success and impact of the programme: this we have called the 'Hampden effect'.

Arrival

Participants entered the stadium via the famous steps that stand in front of Hampden Park, and from which the whole stadium can be viewed. Walking up the steps provided an immediate visual and physical reminder that they were coming to play football at Hampden Park. As a member of staff said, 'People are passionate about it … going there and the atmosphere in Hampden, even just walking up the steps.'

The memories stirred by approaching the stadium created a sense of positive anticipation. On entering the venue, participants and their families or carers were directed by staff to the onsite cafe as the main meeting point. That short walk and the cafe itself are full of images of famous moments, players and teams in Scottish football. All the images and national football memorabilia elicited memories of watching and attending national games, and for a couple of the men, recollections of playing for professional teams at the stadium. One participant remembered visiting Hampden in the past and was surprised by how much the stadium had changed: 'A few times my football has taken me on trips to Hampden so I was aware of this when I came to this. But the first time I came back I looked at it and I couldn't believe it. What a change! It's not what I remember and it's still not what I remember.'

Meeting in the cafe created a central point for all participants, supporters and carers to gather and relax prior to the football session. A volunteer commented on the importance of the pre-session socializing: 'The guys turn up early, you see them over there sitting chatting. It's getting out of the house, coming along and having a bit of a laugh.'

The changing rooms

After leaving the cafe, everyone walked further down into Hampden to the warm-up pitch and changing rooms. The walk was confusing for some as occasionally a different route was taken and all the corridors looked the same, which could become disorientating. This proved an issue for both the players and their families with two spouses stating that, 'We stayed upstairs just for a wee chat the last time and then we got lost.'

The changing rooms were close to the warm-up pitch and provided a space for pre- and post-match 'banter' to enhance the social connections and time spent with other participants. One volunteer spoke of the camaraderie in the changing rooms acting as a leveller: 'I don't think I heard the words Alzheimer's, dementia or anything in the three hours we kicked a ball about. We had a brilliant laugh, everybody, and that's the nice bit.'

The changing rooms were a space for talking about the players who had graced them in the past. One participant spoke of how he had been in those changing rooms many times during his playing days saying: 'It really has [changed] with all the input from the Scottish Football Association and all that. It really has changed quite dramatically and all for the better. It's a big stadium now and it leaves people with the memories.'

Within the changing rooms, the men put on the kits of the teams who had competed in the Glasgow Cup. The kits prompted many memories, and the physical act of changing into the strip within the national stadium seemed to fill the men with confidence. Their demeanour altered from visible apprehension to pride and confidence as they emerged from the changing rooms with heads held high and chests puffed out. The changing rooms, as communal places to put on the team strips of choice, were integral to the sessions held at Hampden Park. This is one key difference to walking football sessions held at other leisure locations where participants tend to arrive ready to play and leave immediately after the session.

A sense of belonging was fostered through donning the kits. Through interviews with families and staff, it was clear that the physical act of wearing them facilitated social interactions between participants as well as embodied memories (memory based in bodily experiences) and reminiscence. A 'Hampden effect' akin to Carone et al.'s (2016) 'Notts County effect' was evident, with a sense of pride engendered through playing in the kit of a professional club. The enhanced embodied experiences encouraged via the physical and social opportunities were of particular importance to the men. Other research into generic walking football supports these findings, suggesting that sessions can evoke a feeling of being young again and creating the positive impact of lifting the mood of participants (McEwan et al. 2019). The act of changing into the kit and having 'normal football banter' in the changing rooms also added to the sense of belonging to the group. The men were no longer viewed as men living with dementia. One volunteer recounted the words of one man in the changing rooms who said he used to go to the pub with his friends, but after his diagnosis he no longer felt part of that group as they now did not know how to talk to him. However, at the football he was just 'one of the lads again'. This, coupled with the sense of belonging to a team, highlights the impact the setting of the changing room can provide: a private space and moment for the men to be together with the group of people they were fostering relationships and sharing experiences with.

The pitch

The stadium's main indoor warm-up pitch was used for the walking football. It is next to the tunnel that leads out to the main pitch, and it provided a private and safe location as only participants and staff could access it. This contrasts with many pitches located in community leisure spaces which can be busy and noisy and potentially disorientating for a person living with dementia. As the daughter of one participant reflected: 'I'm trying to think would he be as comfortable if it was outside, in the cold and everybody walking by. I don't know … I don't think he would do it outside, especially as it's nearing the winter and it's getting colder.'

The positive impact seemed to go beyond those who actively played in the sessions. The spectators' area allowed for the involvement of people who were unable to play due to poor health. In particular, one care home resident who was an avid football supporter attended every session as he liked 'watching … and cheering … I come with my mate'.

The programme organizers recognized that a safe spectating area added to the atmosphere at the sessions. Families and supporters cheered on the men, which also contributed to the sense of camaraderie among the players. While the original plan of the programme included offering breaks to family members or carers, the seating area proved popular. It provided some family members with insights into the men's past lives, as this daughter explains: 'Seeing a whole new side to my dad. Because at the time I was born, he had already given up football. So I knew he had played football … but knowing it and actually seeing it and seeing how much he loves it, I actually really like to just sit and watch him and take hundreds of photos.'

The main stadium

At the break in each session, the group had access to the stadium to cool down and take photos. Men pointed out to each other where they had sat at matches, with one man highlighting the corner he always stood at when on duty as a policeman on match days. This setting therefore helped to build the social aspect of the programme, with the familiarity of the stadium bringing a level of comfort for the men and starting conversations.

Photographs of the stadium provided tangible artefacts for the players to take away after the session to share with family and remind them of playing at Hampden Park. This was illustrated by one family member who said: 'When we go over to visit [his] son over in Atlanta, he was showing him photos saying, look, I go to play the walking football at Hampden.'

The care home that brought some men to the sessions used the photographs as part of their weekly planner, as recounted by this staff member: 'So it says on it … there'll be the walking football and they'll go to that and they'll go back to it … and they'll get a wee reminder about the football.'

A place of celebration

Player of the day awards were presented at each session, with the recipient keeping the trophy as a memento. The awards recognized their contribution and helped promote a positive sense of self-identity and pride, with men telling their families about their successes. For example, one man stated that: 'Today in particular is very special, obviously, you know. That's very nice, so I'll get my wife to frame this [medal] and put it above our bed.' An important consideration for people living with dementia, which can often be overlooked, is the creation of new memories. For the participants and families in this study the experience of playing in a place where many of their heroes had played created special new memories which they could share.

The Scottish Football Museum at Hampden Park was the setting for the end of the programme prize-giving ceremony. The event began with a tour of the museum, which all the participants enjoyed – for example, one man said: 'Just take today – that was a nice surprise today.'

One man found a picture of himself on the wall in the museum during his playing days which he showed great pride over, and this enabled conversation about famous players from that era. The prizes, photographs with special guest footballers and the tour celebrated the participation of players and provided them with mementos they could take away to share and keep.

Learning from the programme

The Dementia-Friendly Walking Football programme held at Hampden Park provided a clear insight into the importance of place in the creation of meaningful experiences and embodied memories for people living with dementia.

To enable participation in such leisure activity, those organizing opportunities must provide support and information in formats accessible to people living with dementia and carers – for example, detail on travel and accessing the venue, what to expect on arrival and during the session. Carers and supporters also need the means, such as time and transport, to support the engagement of those for whom they are caring. The flexibility of options available to carers was valued, with the opportunity to have a separate space in the cafe, to spectate or to leave Hampden Park. The sessions supported carers to use the time as they wished. Providing flexible support or time away is crucial if carers are to feel enabled to benefit from such opportunities too.

What we have described as the 'Hampden effect' need not be solely limited to Hampden Park. Sessions can be embedded within professional football club settings where there exist several key elements, such as those highlighted at Hampden. For example, using a cafe as an area to encourage socialization, perhaps using football memorabilia to stimulate conversation and interactions and incorporating features such as taking team photos, providing team kits and having a celebration event with people from the football community. This format will help promote sports within clubs and communities aimed specifically at people living with dementia.

The expertise of Alzheimer's Scotland in organizing events for people living with dementia and their families contributed to the success of the programme, as did their willingness and ability to make adaptations to the programme when required. Key components of success included geographical accessibility with local transport links, support from the venue (such as staff providing extra wayfinding signage or escorting where needed) and skilled coordination from organizers who were familiar with the needs of participants living with dementia. The sessions also required the sports coaches and volunteers to help design and facilitate the walking football, and to make slight adjustments when required – for example, the warm-up sessions' instructions were simplified and adapted to minimize the reliance on short-term memory.

There is a need to develop protocols that maximize the benefit of taking part for participants. For instance, in these sessions participants benefited from the inclusion of opportunities to foster connections and social interactions with others (in the cafe and changing rooms, and through seeing and discussing football memorabilia before and after the session). It was also important that participants and their carers felt comfortable, safe and welcome at sessions, knowing that it was organized by people familiar with their needs. A key aspect of this relates to filling the knowledge and skills gaps among coaches and volunteers about how best to coordinate and modify sports for people living with dementia. Further research is required into how clubs and charity organizations might modify sports and the spaces within which these take place to include people living with dementia and their carers. Enabling the participation of people living with dementia in sport can counter the cultural and social barriers individuals face, and help to address the negative stereotyping of dementia, through reframing people living with dementia as people actively engaged in their communities.

The influence of the Covid-19 pandemic on the provision of walking football at Hampden Park

During spring 2020, Covid-19 restrictions meant contacts, such as those described above, along with almost all community support for everyone, including those affected by dementia, were paused. We now know that people living with dementia were hugely, perhaps disproportionately, affected by Covid-19, and the measures taken to reduce its transmission (Giebel et al. 2021; Roach et al. 2021).

Alzheimer Scotland staff and volunteers were able to stay in touch with some programme participants either through one-to-one support or an online activity cafe (with support from the digital team at Alzheimer Scotland). For several months, staff were also able to personally deliver or post out themed activity packs (football, gardening, art and crafts). The online groups (football memories, jukebox music, movie memories) were supported by volunteers and staff from Glasgow Life (the operating name of Culture and Sport Glasgow). The community programmes, including football, have now been restarted, both by Glasgow Life and Alzheimer Scotland, and are in a more regular format.

So what does this mean in practice?

For those supporting or enabling the involvement in leisure of people living with dementia

We hope that the findings from this project will be useful to those planning dementia-friendly walking football sessions and contribute valuable insights about venue and place.

- Host sessions in a geographically accessible location with good local transport links.
- Display football memorabilia and artefacts to provide visual orientation and cues to promote and support social interactions. Providing club team kits was also found to be helpful.
- Communicate with and provide support to families and supporters before and after each session. Offer opportunities for families to have time to themselves during sessions, but also a safe sitting area to spectate.
- Provide welcoming visual signage and/or staff to support people find their way within the venue.
- Offer opportunities to take photographs and celebrate participation.

For people living with dementia or their informal or family carers

- Places – whose primary purpose is to offer sport and physical activity – can also provide spaces well suited to socialization and a wide range of social activities. These can be beneficial for family carers as well as people living with dementia.

Acknowledgements

We would like to thank the staff and volunteers at Alzheimer Scotland, Hampden Stadium and Sports Clinic for their support.

References

Carone, L., Tischler, V. and Dening, T. (2016) Football and dementia: A qualitative investigation of a community-based sports group for men with early onset dementia, *Dementia*, 15(6): 1358–76.

Eime, R.M., Casey, M.M., Harvey, J.T. et al. (2015) Participation in modified sports programmes: A longitudinal study of children's transition to club sport competition, *BMC Public Health*, 15(1): 649.

Farina, N., Rusted, J. and Tabet, N. (2020) The effect of exercise interventions on cognitive outcome in Alzheimer's disease: A systematic review, *International Psychogeriatrics*, 26(1): 9–18.

Football Association (2018) *Walking Football: Laws of the Game.* Available to download from: http://www.thefa.com/news/2018/oct/08/walking-football-revised-laws-of-the-game-081018 (accessed 17 May 2022).

Giebel, C., Cannon, J., Hanna, K. et al. (2021) Impact of COVID-19 related social support service closures on people with dementia and unpaid carers: A qualitative study, *Aging & Mental Health*, 25(7): 1281–8.

Jenkin, C.R., Eime, R.M., Westerbeek, H. et al. (2016) Are they 'worth their weight in gold'? Sport for older adults: Benefits and barriers of their participation for sporting organisations, *International Journal of Sport Policy and Politics*, 8(4): 1–18.

Jenkin, C., Hilland, T. and Eime, R. (2018) *Walking Basketball Programme: Evaluation Report for Basketball Victoria.* Available at: https://uhra.herts.ac.uk/bitstream/handle/2299/20331/Jenkin_Hilland_Eime_2018_._Basketball_Victoria_Walking_Basketball_Evaluation_Report.pdf (accessed 10 May 2022).

Kiuppis, F. (2018) Inclusion in sport: Disability and participation, *Sport in Society*, 21(1): 4–21.

Lamb, S.E., Sheehan, B., Atherton, N. et al. (2018) Dementia and physical activity (DAPA) trial of moderate to high intensity exercise training for people with dementia: Randomised controlled trial, *British Medical Journal (online)*, 361: k1675.

McDermott, O., Charlesworth, G., Hogervorst, E. et al. (2019) Psychosocial interventions for people with dementia: A synthesis of systematic reviews, *Aging & Mental Health*, 23(4): 393–403.

McEwan, G., Buchan, D., Cowan, D. et al. (2019) Recruiting older men to walking football: A pilot feasibility study, *Explore*, 15(3): 206–14.

Roach, P., Zwiers, A., Cox, E. et al. (2021) Understanding the impact of the COVID-19 pandemic on well-being and virtual care for people living with dementia and care partners living in the community, *Dementia*, 20(6): 2007–23.

Russell, C. (2020) Because life's there: Understanding the experience and identity of people living with dementia in the context of leisure and fitness centres. Unpublished PhD thesis, University of Worcester.

Sirven, N. and Debrand, T. (2008) Social participation and healthy ageing: An international comparison using SHARE data, *Social Science & Medicine*, 67(12): 2017–26.

van Alphen, H.J., Hortobágyi, T. and van Heuvelen, M.J. (2016) Barriers, motivators, and facilitators of physical activity in dementia patients: A systematic review, *Archives of Gerontology and Geriatrics*, 66: 109–18.

Watchman, K. and Tolson, D. (2015) *Football Reminiscence for Men with Dementia in a Care Home: A 12-Week Pilot Study in Scotland*. Final report. Hamilton, Scotland: University of the West of Scotland. Available at: https://www.learningdisabilityand-dementia.org/uploads/1/1/5/8/11581920/football_reminiscence_final_report.pdf (accessed 31 May 2022).

Watson, N.J., Parker, A. and Swain, S. (2018) Sport, theology, and dementia: Reflections on the sporting memories network, UK, *Quest*, 70(3): 370–84.

14 The online leisure environment

Shirley Evans and Jane Twigg

Summary

Many aspects of our lives are carried out online, and this is increasingly the case. By online we mean the use of computers to access the internet to take part in activities such as work, learning or leisure. Online environments include websites, email, social media such as Facebook and webinar platforms such as Zoom. Online environments can help support the continuation of activities and interests. They can also offer opportunities for new leisure activities. However, there is limited research on the benefits and barriers of online environments as a location for leisure for people living with dementia. Online leisure activity can open up opportunities for access to exercise, singing, arts and heritage and socializing. Jane Twigg, a person living with dementia, describes how she uses technology to access her leisure activities. This helps her to be independent, access support, pursue her interests and live well. There is concern for those who do not have the technology or who are unable to use the technology. Gender, ethnicity, education levels, age, disability and cost can all play a role in whether someone has access to online environments. People living with dementia are often not included in the design and development of online environments or the activities that take place in them. Talking to people about what they want and offering support founded on good relationships can help everyone focus on the purpose of the use of technology. It will enable people to feel safe and comfortable online. This can help foster connections and links to communities. Recommendations for how people can be supported to use online environments include aligning activity to the person's wishes and interests, and including someone, such as a family member or people in the community, to contribute to enabling the person to find and access the online opportunity that is their preference.

About the authors

Shirley Evans has worked in the area of technology and inclusion for over 25 years. More recently she has been carrying out research into post-diagnostic support for people living with dementia. This chapter draws together these two strands.

Shirley completed this chapter alongside Jane Twigg, a woman living with dementia (and a co-editor of this book). Shirley and Jane discussed the subject matter together and agreed the broad themes and topics for inclusion. Jane completed her section of the chapter to illustrate how the online environment as a location for leisure plays a part in her life, highlighting the features of greatest significance.

Introduction

Technology is changing rapidly and increasingly becoming essential to all aspects of our lives, including work, education, government services and leisure. This is related to the expansion of the internet whereby everyone can be digitally connected all the time. To be an active citizen you need to have access to the online environment. Access to information and communications technologies, including the internet, is defined as a basic human right in the United Nations Convention on the Rights of Persons with Disabilities (United Nations 2022).

The online environment for the purposes of this chapter means being digitally connected to the internet by a computer. It can offer opportunities for people living with dementia to access leisure activities in the same way as anyone else, and it might also offer new opportunities or enhance what they already do. Many aspects of daily life, including leisure, which might otherwise be difficult for people to navigate in the physical environment, can be accessed online. It may offer opportunities for independent leisure activity or for participating alongside others. It can also help people organize their leisure activities. Of course, as with offline activities, some online leisure activities may be less beneficial.

There is currently an interest in research and practice on assistive technologies for people living with dementia. This can be defined as technology that is designed to increase the ability of someone to engage in daily tasks and has desired outcomes of improved health and well-being. Thus, the use of technology for people living with dementia is often viewed as therapeutic rather than for enjoyment or leisure. While this does not mean that such technological interventions cannot be meaningful and enhance health and well-being, they might not enhance the sense of citizenship held by individuals. Where there is co-design of technologies alongside people living with dementia this is usually focused on assistive technologies rather than everyday technologies.

This chapter explores the opportunities for leisure activity that an online environment can offer people living with dementia and in doing so considers the interrelationship between social connection and social citizenship. It goes on to examine the barriers to online leisure activity that exist for people living with dementia and therefore to active citizenship. Society presents barriers to online access, including those related to gender, ethnicity, age and education, which in turn can affect purchasing power and knowledge around technology. Even if this layer is negotiated then the design of technologies sometimes presents barriers in terms of age and disability. People living with dementia must engage in what Bartlett (2022) refers to as 'access work' to actually get to the leisure activity. Support from individuals and/or the community may be necessary to overcome these barriers.

Recently published scholarship identified four principles of online social connection: relationships, purpose, technology and community (Evans et al. 2022). In the final section, recommendations are made based on these principles as to how technology and online environments can best be designed, and how people can be supported to experience them as safe, comfortable and enjoyable. The aim of these is to increase people's connections, choices and inclusion when taking part in leisure activities online, and therefore to help them experience active citizenship.

The online imperative

The internet was made publicly available in 1991. In 2005 there were a small number of social media platforms and no smartphones. In 2021, over six out of every ten of the entire world's population had internet access (Internet World Stats 2021). The Covid-19 pandemic fundamentally changed the way people live, work and communicate in an online environment. It impacted on the activities carried out online, and how often and for how long these were done. However, there is no evidence to show that the 'digital divide' between those who have access to technology, and those who do not, which includes people living with dementia, has narrowed.

Connection to the internet is vital for people wanting to engage in society. This includes aspects such as leisure, communication, work and learning and practical aspects such as banking, voting and paying bills. Some leisure activities can only be carried out online, including programming and web design, engaging in online social groups (which may not have a physical counterpart), social media and some forms of gaming. Many leisure activities – for example, flying an aircraft, deep-sea diving and walking – can be mimicked to some extent in an immersive online environment by using simulation technology. A virtual experience can be created, but it will not be able to fully replicate the physical sensory experience of in-person contact, being outside and being with nature. However, for some, the online experience might be the only option for reasons that include disability, access to the location and cost. Some activities can be done online or in the physical environment, and there may be leisure activities where there is a choice as to whether they are done within either setting, such as exercise classes and singing groups. The online environment may enhance engagement in leisure by supporting the organization of activities and social connectedness around interests for example, as well as connecting those who are geographically distanced.

Negotiating the online environment

There are several layers of technology that must be negotiated by people accessing the online environment. Individuals need to have access to the internet, and the quality of this access will depend on a range of factors. Physical access essentially will depend on where someone lives and whether the infrastructure is in place to support connectivity. Questions then arise of whether they want to be online, are permitted to be online and whether they know about and can afford it. Once these issues are negotiated there are a range of types of devices that can enable connection to the online environment. These include a personal computer, laptop, tablet, mobile or smart screen and wearables, which might incorporate a headset and smart glasses, for example. And then individuals need to negotiate the types of online environments for engaging in leisure activity that these devices enable access to: websites, email, apps (often applications for mobile devices), entertainment and gaming platforms, virtual learning environments, webinar and conferencing software, films and TV channels, virtual worlds and augmented reality experiences, social media and other communication channels.

Different devices and methods are used to interact with and navigate online environments – for example, keyboard, touchscreen, stylus, voice activation, facial recognition and brain computer interfaces. The device, platform and the method of interacting with it may depend on what leisure activity is being engaged with. For example, participating in video conferencing will often take place on a tablet using a touchscreen, a laptop or a personal computer with a keyboard. Watching a TV programme may take place on a smart screen – i.e. one offering interactive functions to the user). Someone might not even realize that they are in an online environment because to them it is simply the TV.

This complex landscape can be challenging for anyone, but it may present a range of additional challenges for some people living with dementia, relating to memory, language, communication, attention span, sequencing, problem-solving and comprehension. These aspects can affect people's experiences in an online environment. For example, some people may experience difficulties with perception of digital images of individuals and groups (if offered only from the shoulders up), lack of opportunity to read body language, not being sure of who someone is and the differences between communicating in real time and/or communicating asynchronously. People may have age-related difficulties relating to hearing, sight and manual dexterity. Some of these challenges may change over time or vary from day to day.

In the next section we will present examples of how people living with dementia participate in leisure in an online environment to show that addressing these issues is vital.

Opportunities for leisure in the online environment

People living with dementia go out into the physical environment for the same reasons as anyone else (Bartlett 2022). It is likely, therefore, that they will generally engage in and go online for leisure activities for the same reasons that other people might give for doing so. There is, however, little research around how and why people living with dementia use the online environment for leisure, and the benefits that it affords, particularly in relation to citizenship. The leisure activity might be on an individual basis or as a group, and it may or may not be organized by somebody else. It might be open to everyone or specifically for people living with dementia. In some cases there might be an overlap with a leisure activity and a therapeutic intervention that is specifically aimed at improving health and well-being – for example, joining an online singing group.

Jane Twigg explains why the online environment matters to her for pursuing her leisure interests.

Jane: The online environment is important to me as it helps me to pursue my leisure interests. Leisure activities are life-giving for me.

Firstly, my main way of communicating with friends and family is through email. Email allows me more time to process information than telephone. This is helpful for organizing shared leisure time.

Although I am good at typing, it can be difficult to find the right words, in the right order, so email has the added advantage that I can ask for support when I need to.

However, my main leisure activity is far away from technology. I love to walk! For me, walking is an opportunity to feel like I leave my diagnosis behind and simply live 'in the now'.

The online environment helps me to get more out of my walking.

I recently took part in an ultra-walking challenge (100 km over two days) with two friends. Using email and Zoom were crucial in bringing us together to plan and organize the walk.

During the run-up, I joined the challenge Facebook group. Although posting or commenting myself felt like it might lead to me getting in a muddle, I really enjoyed seeing other people's posts in the build-up to the challenge. It gave me a real sense of belonging and excitement (as well as fuelling my competitive spirit!).

My mobile phone has been a great addition to my walking. I use it to take photographs whenever I walk. This creates a visual diary that I can look back on, but also can share with others without the need for so many words. It also has an SOS function that gives me more confidence to walk alone.

Another leisure activity I enjoy is art. During the 2021 lockdown, I was fortunate to be part of an online creative club run by Rare Dementia Support. I was sent a box of art materials and joined sessions via Zoom.

The facilitators led different themes and it was wonderful because I could take part in the comfort of my own home. I met other people affected by dementia and it felt like a safe space to be a part of.

Although I enjoy art, I can find it hard to know where to start without some support and direction from others. As it was online, it gave me the opportunity to do something that was not available locally. It was great!

I do feel fortunate that I can afford to access the online environment. It adds value to those leisure activities that give me life.

> The online environment helps me to feel like part of a world that is bigger than me. It helps me feel included.
>
> It has also broadened my world more literally, by helping me to build relationships with people who share my interests. These people can support me to actually *be* included, and to take on new adventures and challenges – an important part of who I am.

Jane's experiences illustrate how the online environment functions as a means for supporting her leisure interests. She has a clear purpose for using technology, and it enables her independence, enjoyment and social connection, and therefore contributes significantly to active citizenship.

In the remainder of this section we outline three examples of leisure activity engaged in by people living with dementia. These relate to socializing, singing groups and heritage. These examples have been chosen because they are relatively accessible, popular and came to the fore during the Covid-19 pandemic.

Socializing via social media

There is some literature around the use of social media, mainly by people living with young onset dementia (under 65 years of age). Craig and Strivens (2016) found that in the case of the social networking website Facebook there is much use of the platform in terms of healthcare and peer support, but there is limited mention of its use for leisure, although there may be an overlap. Likewise, Talbot and colleagues (2021) found that people living with dementia used the news and social networking site Twitter largely to maintain a sense of identity, for campaigning and to challenge stigma. However, there is limited literature around the use of social media by people living with dementia over the age of 65, much as would be the case with the general population aged over 65.

We have already seen how Jane uses technology to maintain social connections. Some further examples are described below.

The Zoomettes is a group for women with dementia in the UK and is part of the Dementia Engagement and Empowerment Project (DEEP). The group uses the Zoom platform to connect. Although it was set up as a peer-support group addressing dementia-related issues, leisure activities are discussed including art, exercise, the benefits of having a pet and travelling. Thus it provides social connection and a means of opening up access to leisure activity too.

Dementia Diaries is a UK-wide project that brings together people's diverse experiences of living with dementia as a series of audio diaries. It serves as a public record and a personal archive that documents the views, reflections and day-to-day lives of people living with dementia, with the aim of prompting dialogue and changing attitudes. (Innovations in Dementia n.d.). People use the telephone, mobile phones or other digital devices to record their thoughts and experiences on a regular basis. These recordings are uploaded to a website. While the aim is to improve understanding of the diverse experiences of living with dementia and how communities and services can offer support, it is also an enjoyable exercise for many (Woodall et al. 2016).

Singing groups can provide meaningful activity for people living with dementia (Camic et al. 2011). Little is known about how this translates to the online environment, although the availability of these and uptake indicate that people living with dementia attend and potentially enjoy them. The Covid-19 pandemic saw a rise in interest in participation in online singing groups, and many of these continued after the initial restrictions. Dowson and Schneider (2021) suggest that online singing could be taken up by millions of people living with dementia worldwide as a relatively inexpensive aid to well-being and social inclusion. They also note that it could improve accessibility for those living in remote areas.

Visiting heritage sites, such as historic buildings and ancient landmarks, is one of the most popular activities enjoyed by people living with dementia, as these surroundings often feel safe and familiar (Alzheimer's Society 2021). Visiting a heritage site can improve physical and mental health by helping people keep active (Stewart et al. 2022). Challenges that heritage sites need to overcome include consideration of the progressive nature of dementia, and the need to consider how to support people to continue to enjoy the experience if they can no longer visit in person (Klug et al. 2017). An online experience offers one way to enable this.

After the start of the Covid-19 pandemic many heritage providers increased their offer of online heritage experiences, including those specifically for people living with dementia. One example is through the provision of virtual tours on museum and art gallery websites. Tours can be offered as a click-through experience, in three dimensions, or through the use of a downloadable app. Some heritage sites build on their existing face-to-face tours and cafes by providing online sessions which include virtual tours using video footage.

In this section we have seen examples of how the online environment can be used for leisure, how it complements the physical environment and that it can provide continuity of a leisure activity for people living with dementia.

Barriers to accessing the online environment

Technology used by people living with dementia is generally a means to an end, by which we mean it is not the leisure activity itself but a means to accessing it. In everyday life we understand that there are ways of accessing the physical leisure environment – for example, finding out how and where to buy a ticket, buying a ticket to an event, catching a bus or train and navigating to the destination. There is a similar situation with the online environment. The person needs to identify which environment to access, find a device to access it and then navigate around the system to engage in the leisure activity. Ruth Bartlett (2022) describes this type of effort as 'access work'. Focusing on the experiences of people living with dementia accessing outside spaces using location technologies, such as global positioning system (GPS) devices, Bartlett identifies a need to share the responsibility of the access work. This means the inclusion of someone, such as a family member or people in the community, to enable continued engagement in the leisure activity with the aim of affording independence and active citizenship.

However, even before this access stage, there are barriers to people knowing about the technology. Even if someone knows about it they may be unable to access it because they cannot afford it. Then they might not be able to use it because there is no training or support available. If that is addressed, they might not want to use it, unless there is a very clear purpose and the technology works well. None of the above applies only to people living with dementia of course. Approximately 15 per cent of the world's population has some sort of disability (WHO 2011). Ninety-eight per cent of the top one million websites do not offer full accessibility. It is likely that accessibility is a key barrier to people using the internet, and what follows therefore considers aspects of accessibility and usability for people living with dementia.

It is the law in many countries that online environments must meet international Web Content Accessibility Guidelines (W3C Web Accessibility Initiative 2021). Accessibility standards are inclusive of people with impaired vision, motor difficulties, cognitive impairments or learning disabilities, and deafness or impaired hearing. Some people will experience difficulties in more than one of these areas, and these conditions might change overtime.

Inclusion of people living with dementia in the design of technologies is increasing (Goodall et al. 2021) but not as much as it could. The inclusion has mainly been around technologies specifically designed for people living with dementia and has not yet extended greatly to everyday technologies. However, some everyday technologies are incorporating accessibility features – examples include enabling of different strategies to navigate web content, access to information in text, audio or other formats and provision of opportunities to change the presentation of content according to individual needs or preferences.

Aside from the barriers that are presented to people living with dementia there are characteristics related to the structure of societies which can play a role in whether someone has access to the technology – for example, age, gender, ethnicity and level of education. In the UK virtually all adults aged 16 to 44 were recent internet users (99 per cent) in 2019, compared with 47 per cent of adults aged 75 years and over. However, globally women are 23 per cent less likely than men to use the internet (Broadband Commission 2019). This is due to the limited purchasing power and financial independence of women compared with men. Factors which may influence this include educational levels and expectations held about gender in wider society.

Not being able to afford the technology, not knowing about technologies and not having support will prohibit a person from getting online. Thus there are a range of external factors imposed by society that can prevent a person living with dementia engaging in online activities for leisure, and this hinders their engagement in the community as an active citizen.

Keeping safe online and ethical considerations

The online environment needs to be treated with equal, if not more, caution than the physical environment as it presents additional challenges relating to identity, confidentiality and privacy of information. These can be exacerbated where there are accessibility and usability issues for those with a cognitive impairment, as these issues can make the environment more difficult to use and error more likely. In addition, it is likely that people are more at risk when participating in leisure online as sites will not offer the same protections as banking, government sites and employment platforms. People living with dementia may therefore be at increased risk of, and be concerned about, falling for scams, sharing private information, viewing potentially upsetting information or making unwanted purchases (Tinder Foundation 2016).

These concerns could be addressed through safety features – for example, those that limit access to websites or prevent downloading of spyware (software that collects personal information for nefarious purposes). Difficulties can also be addressed through the involvement of friends or family so that others know what people are doing online, although this does not help someone whose circumstances make them isolated. It may be necessary to learn a person's password, check on lists of contacts and restrict which websites can be accessed.

However, taking precautions such as those described above will mean the person has lost some independence. Consideration must be given to the balance between reducing risk online and maintaining independence when engaging in leisure activities. Conversations about this need to commence at an early stage. This is in line with the idea of 'access work' and 'consciously sharing the responsibility of access work' with others who could be family and friends, neighbours and other community members (Bartlett 2022).

In such circumstances ethical considerations come to the fore. Primarily with assistive technology in mind, some authors (Meiland et al. 2017) note that it is not the technology which presents ethical challenges, but the way it is used. For example, tracking devices may be seen as increasing independence or as keeping watch on someone and invading privacy. Meiland and colleagues suggest this is pertinent to people living with dementia due to possible difficulties individuals may have understanding complex technology and loss of awareness of the presence or purpose of the (assistive) technology. Consideration needs to be given to the implications for potentially vulnerable people and how they can feel safe online. If actions to keep people safe on the internet are not to negatively impact on a person's citizenship, they require a balance of risk that takes the need for autonomy and choice into account. For example, a potential loss of human contact stemming from protection against harm needs to be balanced against the enablement offered by online technology in terms of social connectedness.

Four principles to enable online social interaction

A key aspect of access to online leisure activity for people living with dementia is connectivity – connections with other people and/or opportunities to engage in leisure. Four principles are offered to enable online social connection, based on the work of Evans et al. 2022 and the *Community Makers* project – a network

Figure 14.1 Four principles to enable online social interaction (Community Makers 2021)

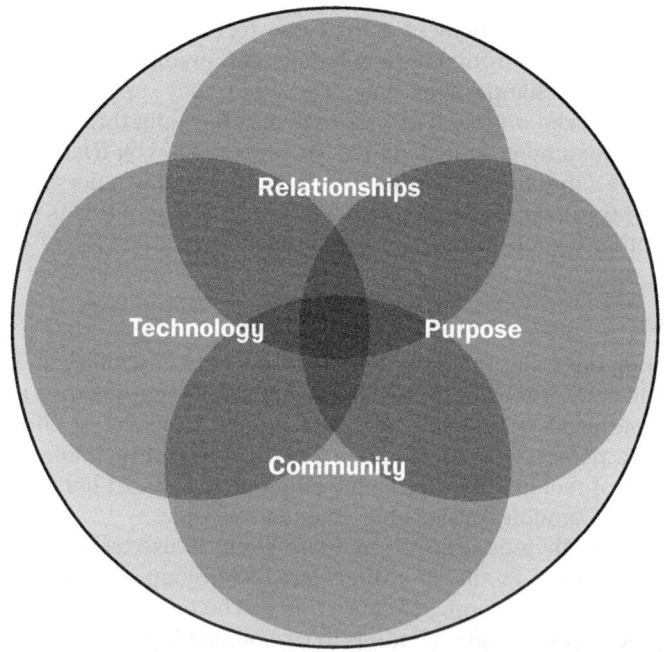

of community groups supporting people affected by dementia, set up to reconnect people during the Covid-19 pandemic. The four principles – purpose, relationships, technology and community – are illustrated in Figure 14.1.

Purpose

People living with dementia who are not familiar with, or are afraid of, technology need a strong and clear reason to overcome perceived barriers. Not everyone will want to join a singing group, for example, so they are unlikely to use
the technology to do this if they are new to both. Purpose is personal and unique
to the individual and there is a role for drawing on trusted relationships, as
discussed further below, to establish what motivates each person. This may be
pertinent for people living with dementia as their condition changes and if they
are not able to communicate their wishes.

If there is a fit between purpose and an individual's preferences, abilities and
activities in using technology, this can foster positive engagement and confidence in contributing as an active citizen. Earlier, Jane clearly described her
purpose for using technology. If technology is used to enhance an activity in
the physical environment, such as the use of email to help organize and support
a walking activity, this can improve health, well-being and enjoyment because
it can offer control, choice and independence.

Relationships

Some people living with dementia may use technology independently and engage in the online environment to enhance their enjoyment of leisure activities, but this might change over time. The additional support needed might come via a formalized outreach programme or informally through friends and neighbours. For example, Jane explains she is supported by friends when writing emails if she cannot find the right words. It may be that a person has family and friends who can support them to get online, but where this is not the case it is a community responsibility to provide that support.

Technology

The technology must suit the individual in terms of accessibility and usability, and it must meet their reason for using it. Giving someone a device may not be enough; people need to be enabled to use it well. However, it should not be assumed that a person with dementia is a novice user of technology. We have seen the range of technologies that Jane employs to support her leisure activities, for example, though her use may change over time.

People living with dementia will be more likely to use technology if everyday versions are made available, rather than technology specifically designed for people living with dementia, because this will be part of normal life and not risk feelings of stigmatization. It stands to reason that if people can be involved in all stages of the conception and design of the technology then it will be easier to use and enhance motivation for use.

Community

Once the technology is in place, and the person feels motivated and able to use it, they can start to connect with others. Even if someone does not want to do this, they are still in a position to connect with leisure opportunities and access services and information, enabling opportunities for active citizenship. For example, Jane Twigg described how technology enabled her to socialize and feel part of the build-up to the ultra-walking challenge.

People may feel more comfortable interacting and initiating conversations in an online community than face to face. Evans et al. (2022) also found that if access to online support and leisure activity is increased, people will benefit from enhanced health and well-being because they will be better able to maintain social networks and connections.

Concluding thoughts

The online environment interweaves with the physical environment and across all aspects of everyday life. Engaging with technology and online environments is a vital part of being an active citizen today and offers opportunities for people living with dementia to engage in leisure. People living with dementia experience all the barriers that others face in terms of accessing online environments, but the situation is exacerbated by the added challenges that dementia brings. People want to engage in leisure and have the right to do so. However, accessing such environments can be denied or require a significant amount of effort, potentially rendering the activity unenjoyable and pointless.

So what does this mean in practice?

For those supporting or enabling the involvement in leisure of people living with dementia

- The further development of everyday technologies to meet the needs of people living with dementia should be prioritized.
- The involvement of people within the development process of the technology is essential. For some, this could become a leisure activity in itself.
- Technology should be designed to be adaptive to meet people's changing situation and needs. People living with dementia would be more independent and have their citizenship strengthened as a result. They would have more choice as to how and when they engaged with leisure activities.

For people living with dementia or their informal or family carers

- Technology can be used to engage with leisure activities. This can help support independence, accessing support and pursuance of interests.
- People should be supported to use online environments through aligning activity to their wishes and interests. Others, such as a family member or people in the community, can contribute to enabling the person to find and access the online opportunity that is their preference.

For researchers

- There should be a focus on research into the use of technology and leisure.
- People living with dementia must play a leading role in this research.

References

Alzheimer's Society (2021) *Risk Factors for Dementia*. Factsheet 450LP. Available at: https://www.alzheimers.org.uk/sites/default/files/pdf/factsheet_risk_factors_for_dementia.pdf (accessed 8 June 2022).

Bartlett, R. (2022) Inclusive (social) citizenship and persons with dementia, *Disability & Society*, 37(7): 1129–45.

Broadband Commission (2019) *The State of Broadband 2019*. Available at: https://broadbandcommission.org/Documents/SOBB-REPORT%20HIGHTLIGHTS-v3.pdf (accessed 6 June 2022).

Camic, P.M., Williams, C.M. and Meeten, F. (2011) Does a 'Singing Together Group' improve the quality of life of people with a dementia and their carers? A pilot evaluation study, *Dementia*, 12(2): 157–76.

Community Makers (2021) *Four Principles to Enable Social Connection*. Available at: https://communitymakers.co/four-principles/ (accessed 6 June 2022).

Craig, D. and Strivens, E. (2016) Facing the times: Young onset dementia, *Australasian Journal on Ageing*, 35(1): 48–53.

Dowson, B. and Schneider J. (2021) Online singing groups for people with dementia: Scoping review, *Public Health*, 194: 196–201.

Evans, S., Harrison, M., Morgan, N. et al. (2022) Community Makers: Report on developing an online toolkit for supporting people with dementia to connect during the pandemic and beyond, *Working with Older People*, 26(2): 140–50.

Goodall, G., Taraldsen, K., and Serrano, J.A. (2021) The use of technology in creating individualized, meaningful activities for people living with dementia: A systematic review, *Dementia*, 20(4): 1442–69. https://doi.org/10.1177/1471301220928168

Innovations in Dementia (n.d.) *Dementia Diaries*. Available at: https://dementiadiaries.org (accessed 6 June 2022).

Internet World Stats (2021) *Usage and Population Statistics*. Available at: https://www.internetworldstats.com/top20.htm (accessed 6 June 2022).

Klug, K., Page, S.J., Connell, J. et al. (2017) *Rethinking Heritage: A Guide to Help Make Your Site More Dementia-Friendly*. London: Historic Royal Palaces.

Meiland, F., Innes, A., Mountain, G. et al. (2017) Technologies to support community-dwelling persons with dementia: A position paper on issues regarding development, usability, effectiveness and cost-effectiveness, deployment, and ethics, *JMIR Rehabilitation and Assistive Technologies*, 4(1): e1.

Stewart, H., Smith, S., Baxter, R. et al. (2022) *Unlock & Revive: The Ingredients needed to deliver Accessible Online Cultural and Heritage Events that bring Positive Benefits to People Living with Dementia*. Edinburgh: Edinburgh Napier University.

Talbot, C.V., O'Dwyer, S.T., Clare, L. and Heaton, J. (2021) The use of Twitter by people with young-onset dementia: A qualitative analysis of narratives and identity formation in the age of social media, *Dementia*, 20(7): 2542–57.

Tinder Foundation (2016) *Dementia and Digital: Using Technology to improve Health and Wellbeing for People with Dementia and their Carers*. Available at: https://www.goodthingsfoundation.org/wp-content/uploads/2021/03/dementia_and_digital.pdf (accessed 6 June 2022).

United Nations (2022) *Convention on the Rights of Persons with Disabilities* (CRPD). Available at: https://www.un.org/development/desa/disabilities/convention-on-the-rights-of-persons-with-disabilities.html (accessed 6 June 2022).

W3C Web Accessibility Initiative (2021) *Cognitive Accessibility at W3C*. Available at: https://www.w3.org/WAI/cognitive/#about-accessibility-for-people-with-cognitive-and-learning-disabilities (accessed 6 June 2022).

Woodall, J., Surr, C., Kinsella, K. and Bunyan, A.-M. (2016) *An Independent Evaluation of 'Dementia Diaries*. Leeds: Leeds Beckett University. Available at: https://dementiadiaries.org/wp-content/uploads/2016/09/Dementia-Diaries-Final-Report-September-2016.pdf (accessed 6 June 2022).

World Health Organization (WHO) (2011) *World Report on Disability 2011*. Available at: https://www.who.int/teams/noncommunicable-diseases/sensory-functions-disability-and-rehabilitation/world-report-on-disability (accessed 6 June 2022).

Afterword

Chris Russell and Karen Gray

In the foreword by Jane Twigg and in this book's first chapter we set out a challenging vision. Our aims were to encapsulate an understanding of leisure within dementia as life-enhancing, to contest the injustice that opportunity to enjoy leisure is not open to people living with dementia as of right, and to introduce theories of dementia and leisure that can be incorporated within practice, research, professional education and in everyday life, so that this vision might be realized.

We are grateful to all the book's authors; they have risen to this challenge and exceeded it. They have introduced a range of novel concepts, such as an exciting framework for celebrating life and creating meaningful and connecting moments, or the idea of 'third places' as a way of understanding how leisure activities within informal public spaces might foster relationships between participants and a sense of community. They have taken readers to settings ranging from sports centres and arenas to museums, galleries and online environments. They have described activities as diverse as quizzes, singing groups and taking a holiday. These contexts and pastimes have been presented in ways that illustrate convincingly that leisure can and must form part of everyday life for people with dementia.

The arguments themselves create further momentum. What might readers achieve now through acting upon the ideas and recommendations on offer? Might there be a need for a companion edition to this book that showcases this innovation? We are very aware that there are gaps in the collection. We highlighted a number of these at the outset and are hopeful that this book might now act as a springboard to remedy some of them. For example, the volume's authors are drawn from across the UK, Canada and USA. However, there is a pressing need to consider the scholarship of researchers and the experiences of people affected by dementia from other countries, and particularly across the Global South, so that we can all benefit from differing perspectives on leisure that result from geography or culture. There is an opportunity also to explore important intersectional issues in greater depth, examining further how aspects of identity and social structure impact on or relate to experiences of leisure and the everyday. We continue to be excited by the involvement of people living with dementia in activism of all kinds, and using leisure to do so, whether advocating for the rights of people with the condition, challenging or 'resisting' stigma or in 'quieter' forms such as craftivism (DEEP 2022). Environmental and climate emergency is the greatest challenge we currently face as a society, and we would particularly welcome the further engagement of scholars into how this relates to ideas of leisure in the context of a condition such as dementia.

A word on the role of Jane Twigg as one of three editors. Jane's introduction set out how she went about her work. This was immersive, with drafts of summary chapters scrutinized and critical feedback offered. The editors worked together as a team to ensure that Jane's vision for the book was maintained. Being an editor living with dementia presented challenges for Jane, including grappling with large amounts of text. However, the benefits are clear to see – a book about dementia, covering an essential element of everyday life, co-edited by a person with lived experience of dementia. Our call is for more of this. We would like to see more books being written in this way.

Thus, while we hope that you have enjoyed the book and that you have found in it learning that you can apply constructively, there remains more to do. This is the start of something that must continue. We therefore conclude with a call for more research, for the incorporation of these ideas within professional education, and for well-informed practice that can achieve what Jane Twigg has advocated: leisure that is life-affirming for everyone living with dementia, at whatever their stage of life, right across the world.

References

Dementia Engagement and Empowerment Project (DEEP) (2022) *Dementia Craftivists.* Available at: https://dementiacreatives.org.uk/dementia-craftivists/what-is-craftivism/ (accessed 9 January 2023).

Index

Page numbers in italics are figures; with 't' are tables.

01 14

J